STROKE

STROKE
A Doctor's Personal
Story of his Recovery

By Charles Clay Dahlberg, M.D.
and Joseph Jaffe, M.D.

W·W·NORTON & COMPANY·INC·
NEW YORK

Copyright © 1977 by Charles Clay Dahlberg and Joseph Jaffe
Published simultaneously in Canada by George J. McLeod Limited,
Toronto. Printed in the United States of America.

Library of Congress Cataloging in Publication Data

Dahlberg, Charles Clay.
    Stroke: a doctor's personal story of his recovery.

    1. Cerebrovascular disease—Biography.   2. Dahlberg,
Charles Clay. I. Jaffe, Joseph, 1924–   joint author.
II. Title. [DNLM: 1. Aphasia—Personal narratives.
2. Cerebrovascular disorders—Personal narratives.
WL340 D131s]
RC388.5.D33 1977   616.8′1′09 [B]   77–414
            ISBN 0 393 08720 4
            1 2 3 4 5 6 7 8 9 0

For Jane, John and Jim
—C.C.D.

For Anna C. Jaffe and, in memoriam, Julian F. Jaffe
—J.J.

Contents

Preface and Acknowledgments

There are stories which cannot be told too often. They concern universal experiences of the human predicament. One of these is a possibility that each of us faces: a disaster within the brain which demolishes our language ability. Each account of this experience contributes a sharply defined point of view, and expands our knowledge of it.

For the account to be firsthand, the storyteller must survive the experience. He must also remember it, and recover to the point of being physically able to tell the tale. Finally, he must want to tell it. Given all these constraints, personal accounts of language loss from brain disease are understandably rare, and nearly improbable if the protagonist is a physician. That he is also a psychiatrist with specialized training in psychoanalysis renders this account unique.

Based on hospital admissions, five to six hundred thousand people in the United States suffer a stroke each year, and a majority do survive. Two-and-a-half-million stroke victims are alive in America today. Due to vicissitudes of medical reporting, all the above figures are probably lower than actual figures would show.

Of all surviving stroke victims, about ten percent are virtually unimpaired, forty percent have a mild residual disability, forty percent require special daily care, and ten percent need institutional care.

Statistically practically nobody has a stroke before age

9

thirty-five and the incidence increases with age. Therefore, many patients have children and possibly grandchildren. There is no way of estimating the cost of caring for all these stroke victims outside of the hospital, but exclusive of physicians' services and non-hospital care, the cost is estimated at $1.2 billion a year. This makes a stroke the single most costly disease in this country. (Patients live longer and require more care than cancer and heart disease victims.) Add to this the financial and emotional costs of this kind of prolonged stress on families of the out-of-hospital patient. Motivation for recovery from stroke can be greatly influenced by the attitudes of family, friends, employers, physicians, and self. It is to these persons that this book is addressed.

The brain does many things: it sees, hears, feels, smells, and tastes; it controls our movements, our internal organs, our hormones, and it is the seat of consciousness. Certain special parts of the brain control the language mechanism. For reasons which we will explain, about half of all stroke victims run the risk of *aphasia*, a language disorder which results from brain damage. We emphasize this particular symptom because of our interest in communication and also because it is the most mysterious and poignant effect of a stroke.

This is a technically accurate but easily understood account of how a stroke damages the brain to produce aphasia. We have tried to abandon medical jargon. However, we have found that translating medical jargon, which is a kind of shorthand, can frequently become quite cumbersome, so in some cases we use it after defining it once.

Language is the most complex ability that human beings have, and it is small wonder that we know so little about it. We prefer to present our painfully meager knowledge in naked form; in plain, everyday English when we can. One can even hope that the removal of the "Emperor's clothes" will stimulate some intelligent layman to think about the problem and make some useful suggestion which would freshen our clinical approach. Language, thought, and communication are everyone's business. New concepts are desperately needed.

How does the brain produce language? By comparison, the problems of landing a man on the moon or cracking the genetic code are about as complicated as skimming a flat stone off the surface of a pond. Nobody knows how the brain creates language. If that is what distinguishes man from the apes, then the brain mechanisms underlying our humanity remain shrouded in mystery.

One major casualty of the traditional separation between science and the humanities, the "two cultures" of C. P. Snow, has been our knowledge of the brain mechanisms underlying language. The situation is comparable to a criminal investigation in which experts in the police crime lab fail to communicate with the detectives questioning the witnesses in the case. The separation has been nearly total until now; however, there have been new rays of hope recently. Linguists and medical researchers are at last learning how to communicate with each other, and this is precisely the conceptual bridge we require in order to understand aphasia. In order to hasten this synthesis, we do not simply tell Clay Dahlberg's story and offer the standard medical explanations. We also devote chapters to the following questions: What is language?; Is it learned or inherited?; What is the distinction between language ability *per se* and the various ways in which it contacts the minds of other human beings—for example, speech, writing, sign language of the deaf, and body language? Finally, what brain mechanisms underlie it?

It is barely a century since the site of language ability was first tracked down to one side of the brain. The idea was revolutionary at the time, yet is now a basic principle of neurology. One cannot escape the feeling that other such principles may now be staring us in the face, begging to be recognized. Fresh observations are required, and the best source are the self-reports of recovered aphasics, especially those with specialized knowledge relevant to the problem.

Although the book was jointly authored, the writing task

was split: Clay Dahlberg is responsible for Chapters 1, 2, 8, 9, 10, and 11—the journal of his illness; Joe Jaffe for Chapters 3, 4, 5, 6 and 7 which are a somewhat tutorial commentary on Dahlberg's story. We refer to each other by our given names which we use when talking to one another. Since the writing was done independently, but with frequent consultations between the authors, personal acknowledgments will follow.

I thank my doctors and nurses (except one). My doctors, Jim Leland and my neurologist, are endeared for their devotion to me. In the book, I call Jim Leland only by his last name to avoid confusion with my son Jim. My neurologist preferred not to be identified: "I avoid publicity." I refer to him as Cicero Zeugma. My special nurse, Frank, was especially supportive. There were many others behind the scenes in the hospital who helped. Most importantly, they did not treat me as an "object." I was never in any way humiliated. When I needed help, I received it.

Others who helped in preparing the book are Dr. Richard S. Benua, Dr. Henry Selby, and Frank Taylor. Also, I thank the many doctors who conferred with me at hospitals in Copenhagen, as well as the late Dr. George Wise, and my ophthalmologist Dr. Marvin Gillman. And of course, I thank Mercedes Barry, who not only transcribed many of my dictated tapes, but offered me comfort and cheer, as did too many of my friends to mention.

Ruth Duell, who encouraged me with the book, offered us her home for writing, and edited some of the manuscript, has my undying appreciation for these and other remarkable courtesies she and her deceased husband, Charles, extended.

I must mention my patients, especially those four who wrote sections at my request. Frequently they did so under great stress. One said, "The whole thing is upsetting to me. Perhaps *you* should write an essay about what happens to your patients when they are asked to write how they feel about your illness." Perhaps I shall, but I hope I don't get too many more calls for that.

It must be obvious to anyone who reads the book that it could never have been written without my wife Jane. Not only did she give me moral support and prodding, but she did a great deal of proofreading, typing, rewriting, and reordering of paragraphs, sentences and thoughts. Aphasic dictation is, after all, aphasic.

—Charles Clay Dahlberg, M.D.

I am indebted to many colleagues who offered advice and criticism, and often disagreed with specific interpretations. The year of Clay's stroke, Drs. Samuel Anderson and Jason Brown ran a neurolinguistic seminar in the Department of Communication Sciences which I direct at the New York State Psychiatric Institute. Naturally, Clay's symptoms were discussed and clarified there. Drs. Martha Denckla and Edwin Weinstein were most helpful, and Dr. Daniel Stern contributed the developmental focus which underlies the concept of imitative brain mechanisms. Professor Alex Heller helped us think about Clay's mathematical problems. Dr. Lawrence Kolb, then Chairman of the Department of Psychiatry at Columbia University, is unique in encouraging interdisciplinary projects such as this among his professors.

The ideas and influence of Drs. Morris Bender, Hans Lukas Teuber, Davis Howes, Norman Geschwind, David Rioch, Harold Goodglass, Edith Kaplan, Warren McCullough, Max Fink, John Rainer, Kenneth Altschuler, Robert Rieber, Rita Rudel, Marcel Kinsbourne, Lois Bloom, Beatrice Beebe, Maureen Dennis, Joseph Bogen, and Harry Whitaker suffuse the test.

Earlene Stundis typed the manuscript with skill and intelligence. Carl MacDougall, then on the Youth Opportunity Program in our laboratory, transcribed thousands of words of ·

disorganized aphasic speech, and then classified and timed them. This aspect of the book was partially aided by a general research support grant from the New York State Psychiatric Institute.

My wife, Nora, edited continuously and tried to keep the technical writing intelligible and human. She also acted as a coolheaded moderator in the sometimes difficult task of collaborating with a sick friend whose communication with me, during the first year of his convalescence, suffered from the very difficulties we are attempting to describe.

—*Joseph Jaffe, M.D.*

STROKE

Chapter 1 "In the beginning was the word . . ."

Chapter 9 "That was the true Light . . ."
—The Gospel, according to St. John
1611, King James Version

1

The Incident

Medically, a stroke is called a cerebrovascular accident (*cva*), but to the person who has one, it is a "stroke" because it is like being hit on the head with a blunt instrument. You feel faint and may have convulsions or vomit. Your limbs are weak or helpless and perhaps numb, and if you remain conscious, your thinking is unclear. You may have a severe headache or feel no pain whatsoever. Above all, it is the suddenness of the episode which makes "stroke" the common term.

On Tuesday night, April 24, 1973, I came home from teaching about 9:00 P.M. I talked to my wife Jane, who was preparing to retire early, and then went downstairs and chatted awhile with my son Jim. A meal had been left for me on the dining table, and I took along a newspaper to read; my custom when eating alone. At the first bite I choked and coughed and my vision became hazy. This seemed to clear up in a few minutes and I could read the paper again. Very shortly however, I choked and coughed again. Although my vision was all right this time, the attack seemed worse and I felt weak. When I tried to call for help I could not. I knew what I wanted to say but the words wouldn't come out. I felt in my mouth for any food left there but could find none. I used my left hand because my right hand seemed to be hanging down a bit—weak, but not paralyzed. At this point I knew I had suffered a stroke; as a doctor I recognized the symptoms.

Fortunately, my son Jim came down to the dining room then, and I must have looked odd to him. As I remember, he said something like, "If you're goofing around it doesn't seem funny." When I didn't reply he seemed frightened. He asked if I had food in my mouth; I wasn't sure (the sensation in my mouth and face was affected). He probably saved my life by opening my mouth and pulling out a piece of meat. He's bright and a doctor's son, so he saw I had been eating and made a quick decision. He called for Jane.

Jim's version: When it first occurred I was shocked, but not really. I had known for a few weeks that Dad was seeing physicians often, had had urine samples, etc., so he was doing more than the usual routine check-ups. The night of the stroke I was not totally aware of the seriousness of what had occurred; in fact, I was painting a cabinet while he was eating dinner, and I came in to chat. He did not respond to me and I thought he was "playing spastic"—a comic routine of his. I got cross and demanded that he stop, and it was only then that I knew this was real. He was choking and drooling, and his face was slightly distorted. I pulled some ham out of the back of his mouth and felt for more. I then called my mother, and while she was trying to get him to respond I went back to painting, trying all the while not to be too anxious.

In Jane's words: When I came into the dining room, Clay was sitting at the table looking at his plate. All he could do when I questioned him was say "ur" and move his hands around. He motioned to the newspaper and I thought he must have read some upsetting news. He then acted as if he were writing and I understood he wanted a pad and pencil. (That was the beginning of a few days of charades while we tried to decipher his sounds and motions. It was most frustrating for him because he could think clearly, but could not communicate in words.) He tried to copy a line from the newspaper unsuccessfully. It was not an important sentence and I had no idea what the trouble was. It was absolutely clear however that there was trouble. I said that I was going to call Dr. Leland (our internist and friend) and Clay nodded. Dr. Leland came as soon as he could but it must have been about twenty minutes since he lived quite a distance away. In the meantime Clay had risen from his chair, climbed one flight of stairs, and sat in his office. He seemed better by the time Dr. Leland arrived. He said a few words to the doctor and was able to write for him.

I remember Leland arriving, looking me over, examining my eyes, and asking me to write. When I couldn't think of anything to write, he suggested, "My arm is all right." I didn't know what he meant until Jane, said, "Write 'my arm is all right,' " and I wrote as clearly as ever.

After the examination and the doctor's unsuccessful effort to get a nurse to stay with me in the middle of the night, I walked up another flight of stairs to my bedroom where Jane and Jim were to take turns watching me. Leland was to return in the morning.

Jane writes: Jim and I helped him undress, but he did most of it himself. Soon after the doctor left, Clay got out of bed twice to look at himself in the mirror. Clearly, he was watching his face to observe what was happening to it. Twice during the night he sat up and I thought he was having a nightmare. He waved his arms around, made noises, and then lay back and slept.

To my surprise I was not particularly uneasy or anxious during the night and had no pain. I slept comfortably except for an uncertain number of times when I felt my mouth twitching uncontrollably.

I have no memory of what I had seen in the mirror Tuesday night, but I did have a hand mirror placed by my bed and discovered on Wednesday morning that the right side of my face had collapsed. Hospital arrangements were made for me; I had no objections and was eager for people to take care of me. An ambulance was called.

I had little trouble getting out of bed on my own and going to the chair the attendants carried me down on. I had some power left in my arms since I clutched the hand mirror (Jane offered to carry it but I didn't want to let go—it allowed me to observe my symptoms), and I picked up a book from a table as I was carried past it. I also grabbed onto the stair rail while being carried downstairs—I didn't feel too secure about being carried. Both arms were in use.

While I was in the ambulance Jane and Jim embraced me to comfort me. I looked at the sky as I went into the hospital and wondered if I would see it again, but I felt no fear. It soon developed that this was my "stroke personality"—without anxiety, confident I would be cared for, a perfect undemanding patient. I later asked Dr. Zeugma, my neurologist, if my lack of anxiety was typical of stroke victims. He replied, "Some have it and some don't."

My only concern at that time was that I might lose my sense of humor from possible brain damage. Humor is what keeps many people going in a world they cannot control. My humor in the past had sometimes been considered "black." In fact, before leaving the hospital I had printed, with great effort, the single word "weedee" on a piece of paper. This was the last word I could write for several days. (I had no doubt then that something in my brain had affected my speaking and writing ability.) "Weedee" was my way of telling Jane, in a "black" humor metaphor, that I had had a stroke. It referred to a neighbor who had also had a stroke; we used to talk to him when we met on the street. He could clearly understand us, but the only word he could ever say was "wee-dee, weedee, weedee." He was a sweet man and we all liked him and felt sorry for him. He died a few years ago. As I wrote down "weedee," I pointed to myself and I think I made an effort to smile.

Jim recalls: During the ambulance ride, one of my most intense reactions developed—crying aloud—something I find very hard to do in front of people. I said to Dad, "Why does it always take something like this to bring us together." (My grandmother's funeral a year before was another instance.) We held each other as best we could in the ambulance. I escorted him through the hospital, finding myself defensive in an almost territorial way whenever the nurses tried to do anything.

In some ways, as a doctor, I reacted as an observer of a patient—me. The night I had the stroke, for instance, I had been teaching a course in psychophysiology—the effect of the mind on the body and vice versa. As an M.D. and a psychoanalyst, I was in a unique position to observe my mind and body interacting, and to follow the course of my illness from its outset. I had never lost consciousness from the stroke.

After eight days in the hospital and a few days of recovery at home, I started, laboriously, to make notes on what I remembered. The above and much of what follows is from notes and dictation, and from my family's memories which they wrote later.

The most damaging effect of my stroke was *aphasia*. The prefix "a" in Greek stands for "without, not, or less than." Two of the common words which everyone knows are *amnesia*, meaning loss of memory, and *anesthesia*, meaning loss of sensation. A third word is *aphasia*. This is, literally, the loss of speech, but not because of some superficial problem with the speech apparatus in the mouth and throat. If you are simply gagged, you can still read, write, and understand speech. In aphasia the language ability underlying all these activities suffers damage. This was the major symptom of my kind of stroke. I had almost complete aphasia the first morning in the hospital. I could neither speak, read, nor write, but I retained some ability to understand what people were saying to me. My nonverbal comprehension was, to the best of my knowledge, unimpaired.

As a psychiatrist, I have been accused of knowing what goes on in peoples' minds, but nothing could be farther from the truth. Every thoughtful person knows that more knowledge creates more questions—not certainty. My knowledge about aphasia did not affect my "stroke personality." Many of us at times think about the possibility of a crippling accident or a situation where we might want to die; doctors however, have access to what it takes to kill themselves, assuming they retain the mental capacity to make such a decision. Fortunately, I had not reached a suicidal state. I was calm, "rational," and for no good reason, convinced that I could beat the aphasia.

Settled in the hospital—intravenous in my arm—and in competent hands, I set about communicating. Modesty is not one of my virtues. I am clever with words and mechanics. Jane had a pad and pencil. I was *going* to communicate. She quickly saw what I wanted and wrote down the alphabet on a pad. Nothing to it. I would point to the letters to form the words I wanted and she would write them down.

I have no memory of what I wanted to say—"cancel patients," "don't worry," "I love you"—because it never got through. (Jane thinks I was trying to spell "martini.") With utter confidence I pointed to each letter and she wrote them down and showed it to me. It was a combination of "A," "I," and "U." She tried to guess what I meant but couldn't. We started again with the same result; I was beaten. Fortunately, my nonanxious stroke personality came to the rescue. I shrugged and gave up.

In terms of my comprehension at that time, I always knew Jane, Jim, Leland, and Zeugma. If someone had said to me, "Who is that?" pointing to Jane, I would somehow have been able to indicate that she was my wife, perhaps with an embracing gesture. This meant that I could comprehend certain simple things despite the fact that I could neither speak, read, nor write.

I am quite sure that I also knew Jane's name although I couldn't say it. If someone asked me to repeat a word I could not do it, but if someone showed me simple objects and asked if I knew what they were, I could nod "yes" or "no" correctly. For instance, I could distinguish between a pencil and a coin. When Zeugma asked me to press against his hands with my hands or feet, I could do that. Complicated directions such as "put your right hand on your left ear and your left hand on your left eyebrow" were impossible for me.

I could, and also did, a brief neurological examination on myself. Clearly this could not be extensive; for instance, I could not test my own reflexes while I had to lie still with the intravenous in one arm. But I knew I could hear well, and from both ears. I could also tell the direction that voices came from. I could feel with my feet, and there was reasonable sensation in my hands because I could feel the difference between the mirror and the book that I had carried to the hospital. I could also feel the sheets and knew they were different from the metal bars on the sides of the bed. I could close my eyes, move my limbs, and I could understand certain commands from the nurses—for example, "Don't move now, we'll lift you onto the bed." When another nurse asked, "Which arm should I put the needle in? Are you right-handed?" I could nod assent. (She therefore put the needle in my left arm so my right arm wouldn't be tied up.)

I squeezed my fingers together but could not really tell whether I was squeezing equally, and then I moved my hands around to see whether I could move the fingers in all directions. It was quite apparent that I could not spread the fingers on my right hand as far as I could on my left hand. There was no doubt, after looking in the mirror, that the right side of my face had fallen and would not move.

I also saw in the mirror that I could close each eye, but did not think to check whether I could wrinkle my forehead. I could close one eye with my hand and test my visual field which seemed good, as good at least as one could tell from this kind of self-examination; certainly there were no obvious blind spots.

I had studied neurology but never practiced it. I knew the tests. I was creative enough to use the materials at hand—I was curious, and to that degree I was creative. That same day both Leland and Zeugma did some tests as they examined me. I remember clearly that at the time I had a Babinski reflex on both feet. If the Babinski, however, was on my left foot, it shouldn't have been there. That was so startling to me that I remembered it, and later thought my memory was again playing tricks with me. To my surprise, when Joe looked at my hospital chart, there it was, "left Babinski for one day."

Later that day I looked at my feet. I couldn't tell my right foot from my left. That puzzled me. When the nurse had put the intravenous needle into me and asked me if I was right or left-handed, I had raised my right hand. Therefore, my left hand was the one with the intravenous. But when I looked down at my feet, I didn't know which was which.

It was a few days later that I asked Jane to call Joe Jaffe, probably by pointing to my head and saying, "Joe." He asked me several questions to determine where I was at, but he could not understand my confusion about my feet and questioned me intensely about it.

Joe writes: When I visited Clay in the hospital my initial reaction was one of sadness. A friend and longtime research collaborator was hurt—not just sick, doctors know too much about sickness to get off that easily—hurt. Jane was present, and since I didn't know her too well, emotions were fairly controlled. Clay and I had been doing research for a decade on the linguistic effects of LSD and Amphetamine. The irony was that he knew, and I knew that he knew, and he knew that I knew that he knew, that one of my original motivations for this research was the problem of aphasia. And now he had it. Fortunately, our collaboration furnished a ready-made format for coping with this tragic encounter. Jointly, we could get interested in a fascinating symptom.

The conversation was quasi-clinical—we discussed his language symptoms—I listened and asked occasional questions. He had difficulty finding appropriate words so there were long pauses. Since I could usually sense what he was driving at I could often supply the missing item, and he nodded assent when it fit. His aphasia was so typical that I hesitated to really examine it. It seemed weird coming from a friend. As a result I completely neglected to ask about arithmetic ability. He called my attention to it weeks later, but at the time of this meeting he might have been unable to count to five or add two plus two had I checked. The trouble is that in order to properly assess any deficit you have to push a patient to the point where they fail at something—test limits, so to speak. This invariably and unavoidably leads to a sudden drop in self-esteem, which Clay didn't need at a time when he was struggling to say the simplest sentence. It's hard to do research on a friend. For example, arithmetic ability had no special bearing on his diagnosis or treatment at the moment, so I suppressed my intellectual curiosity, that is, until he mentioned that he knew his right hand from his left but couldn't tell which foot was which. I admit that grabbed me and he seemed damn curious himself. We were suddenly back to our old collaboration, puzzling over a patient's symptom in the perennial hope of contributing to medical knowledge.

Of course, this time the patient was Clay himself. But I was accustomed to such surprising statements from him, having long been an observer of his reports on LSD therapy, many of which strained credulity. But over the years, as each of his initial reports was verified by other investigators, I'd come to respect his enthusiastic objectivity. So when he described the mysterious right-left confusion, there seemed to be something in the room that was bigger than both of us.

It is interesting that we think of the right-left distinction as an abstract orientation in space; that we know our right from our left sides, generally. Even if a limb is paralyzed or anesthetic you know which side it's on. How could he know his right hand from his left but not his right foot from his left foot? This mystery was to preoccupy us for a year. As I left the hospital I recall thinking that he'd gotten a rotten deal, and feeling glad it was not I. Also, I wondered whether he'd recover to the extent of being able to publish all his experiences with his usual clinical intuition.

I had tried at the time to ask Leland to explain the right-left confusion to me. By pointing and using various motions and facial expressions I was trying to communicate, to learn what was happening to me and satisfy my medical curiosity. He took a piece of paper and drew a diagram of the brain which satisfied me. I now realize I didn't get my question across to him nor did I understand his drawing. It illustrated where the foot nerves come from, and where the speech areas are in the brain.

The rest of the day was vague. Mostly I slept, awakening briefly for the usual hospital procedures of taking my pulse, respiration, and blood pressure, and giving me a few shots. I am sure Jane and Jim were there but I paid little or no attention to them. Mercedes, my friend and former secretary, was my first visitor and I remember her hug and smile. Jane told me later that she burst into tears in the hall.

Jim: At this point I finally realized what I had come close to realizing all year, that this was the first year I had spent being comfortable and open with my parents and with people in general; openness and ease with people had never been one of my traits. Now I was finally realizing how much I enjoyed my father, and we were just starting to get comfortable and open when—bang!—the stroke threw everything off course. It was not a downgrading of emotions but it felt different, and, of course, the stroke made us all distant in a new way, yet closer in another way as well.

And so we had a bond. All the while, Johnny was on Cape Cod; we called him immediately of course, but advised him not to rush down that night, but rather to come soon—which he did. It's too bad that John wasn't able to be around all the time.

Leland ordered private nurses for me, as he explained, mainly to keep the pressure off Jane, and not because of any special care I would need. The night nurse was a nightmare who managed to keep me awake because she either fell asleep or noisily left the room to get something to eat. I made some indication that I wanted Valium to help me sleep because I didn't want to spend my night in a rage at her. I also managed to convey to everyone the next day that I didn't want her back.

When Leland came in the next morning I could see the relief on his face. Although it may have been because he had had a pleasant breakfast, I assumed it was about me. The left Babinski was gone. Zeugma gave me a spinal tap, showed me the clear fluid, and announced that the pressure was normal. I also urinated a small amount to everybody's delight.

People vary in terms of what they want to know about their illness. As a doctor and a "participant observer" I certainly wanted to know everything, and am fortunate that my relations with my doctors and my family made this possible. My daily discussions with Leland, following his examinations, included the frank discussion of all symptoms and their significance as far as recovery was concerned. Jane and our sons also participated in honest and open consideration of all the medical aspects of my stroke.

I myself knew that I was improving for I felt more alert. I glanced at *The New York Times* but couldn't read it. The headlines didn't seem to make sense even though I could see them clearly enough. I think I talked a little with Frank, the morning nurse, who was a complete joy—competent, cheerful, efficient. Jane told me that one of my patients was in desperate shape and I nodded assent to Jane's suggestion that she be referred back to the doctor who had originally recommended her to me.

By this time everybody at the Institute where I teach knew what had happened, and any possibility of keeping my illness a secret was gone. New York City is a small town in the way gossip travels, so I knew that Jane should notify my patients about my illness as soon as possible. I would have liked it kept a secret because it's not very constructive for patients who have long-term relationships with a psychiatrist to know that he has a possibly recurrent illness and is unable to speak. But at that moment someone else would have to deal with them.

My interest in the world was minimal, but I was pleased with Jane and Jim's attention to me, and the news that my other son John, who was out of town, was coming home. I didn't know until later that many of our friends came and sat with Jane while I was sleeping. She kept most of them out of the room except for a few brief visits from close friends.

Although I am not a very social person, I have a good many friends. It is our custom generally, especially among men and women, to kiss on meeting. I remember that when I could first talk, one woman came in and put her face against mine without the usual kiss. I remarked, "It's not catching." I thought this was pretty funny and I repeated it to several other people. It wasn't until about three months later that I realized I must have been pretty unattractive. My face was sagging badly and I was drooling, which happens when the lips won't work properly.

That Thursday night it was decided that I could swallow and they gave me a liquid diet. I was getting hungry so they pulled out the intravenous. I had to be very careful to swallow slowly, but I went rapidly from liquids to a soft and then regular diet. I can't remember ever enjoying food so much, and had a better appetite than I'd had since I was a growing teenager. I think this was a side effect of the cortisone I had been given in order to cut down on excess swelling on the brain.

On the third day after my stroke, Zeugma came in and asked if I understood an article in the newspaper with a headline about the problems of financing medical schools; there were pictures of deans of medical schools. He asked me if I could read it and I nodded. Then he asked what the pictures had to do with the headlines. I somehow indicated I knew they were related—it was a series of charades. Possibly, I pointed to Jane who was a college dean. I knew I couldn't say the word "dean," but he was satisfied that I understood the concepts.

Leland told me that day that he no longer had to see me twice a day but since there was a meeting at the hospital later he would drop by. He also ordered a commode to be placed beside my bed for my use, instead of a bedpan. The doctors thought I would strain less with a commode and therefore not suddenly alter my blood pressure as I might with a bedpan. Unless you are used to it, a bedpan is an uncomfortable way to have a bowel movement. Frank helped me onto the commode and within a few days I could manage alone.

Jane observed: Outwardly the commode was a big, old-fashioned, comfortable chair, like a relic from an ice-cream parlor, and Leland usually sat on it when he talked with Clay, instead of using the usual hospital chairs. It embarrassed me a little but both he and Clay saw nothing odd. Doctors don't get embarrassed about the same things I do.

That night I watched the basketball playoffs on TV and could easily follow the plays. I was improving figuratively, if not literally, by leaps and bounds.

During my remaining days in the hospital my speech continued to improve. On Saturday, an old and very close friend (Sidney) called me. He was a patient in another hospital and he had several funny stories to tell me. I was able to talk well enough to be understood. Frank told me I sounded better than I had yet, and there is no doubt that this was due to the emotion I felt on hearing my friend's voice. So much of the language impulse is emotional. (My ability to write "weedee" on Wednesday morning was also emotionally fueled.)

I have three notes in which I wrote Sidney's name: after one week in the hospital I wrote "Sedeny"; one week later I wrote "Sedney"; three weeks poststroke I wrote "Sidney." I knew the first two were wrong, but not what was wrong with them.

Speech, as it improved, was quite fatiguing and had to be limited to short periods with only one person at a time. It was impossible for me to speak at all with other noises or conversations going on simultaneously. Joe later said it was like a telegram where you pay for every word, and pay you do. The coin is fatigue.

I also shaved with my electric razor that day, which is a good sign—like women starting to comb their hair and put on make-up, it shows a concern for the feelings of others and a pride in your own appearance.

From then on it was all uphill. I slept a good deal. Visitors only stayed for ten to fifteen minutes. This was the time of Joe's visit which was described previously. I think it was the day that I had the brain scan and EEG (Electroencephalogram).

After five days in the hospital Leland warned me that the first days of recovery are the fastest, and that improvement continues much more slowly later. I was happy as a clam and didn't give a damn. Giving a damn came a few weeks later.

Before long I was out of bed in a wheel chair, and sat by the window looking over the river. I gradually learned to eat slowly so I wouldn't cough. I also indulged in one of my favorite vices—reading the racing form. Occasionally, to show my confidence in my judgment I made a small bet. I discovered that I couldn't add or subtract without great difficulty, and could rarely tell whether I had added two single digits correctly or not.

My son, Johnny, arrived and wheeled me around the hall. I told him I had heard one could see a naked girl in the window of an apartment across from one of the hospital rooms ("inside dope" from one of the nurses). We went looking, but had no luck. We did carry on a small conversation, however, about voyeurism, and I was delighted that I could "enjoy" the prospect of a naked girl, as well as share some thoughts with Johnny. It meant that I knew and remembered more complex concepts.

I was starting to get itchy to be out. Leland finally discharged me Wednesday afternoon, the eighth day after my stroke. He and Zeugma agreed that I could go home, but felt I should stay indoors and treat myself as though I were still in the hospital. I could go up and down the stairs once a day. I had to take two aspirins twice a week, later changed to daily doses to diminish blood clotting, and a drug I had started taking the day of the stroke to lower my blood pressure. I was also given a diminishing dose of cortisone for a few days. As I was getting dressed, Leland came back into the room and said, "As for sex, none until you have a clear brain scan." It was the least of my worries at the moment.

That was a glorious day. I started planning all the things I could do with the incredible amount of free time I was going to have. Chores I had put off, museums and galleries to visit, friends I had wanted to meet for lunch—so many joyful things.

It was not until several days later that I realized I simply couldn't do them. I didn't have the mental or physical

Saturday 5/5/73

I have been in good health. ~~Pt~~ Poor
~~exercise~~ ~~diet~~, too much smoking. Routine visit to ~~~~ internist
revealed BP 180/90. ~~B~~ Something of test to ~~~~
unless domenathing turned up. Nothing. Osteophictytes
on neck which ~~some~~ trouble. ~~~~

~~~~ Two or ~~three~~ tronight ~~~~ ~~~~ × 3 wk
albrights to inestright I told head & on arising
in am I have had my have & should down
on arising. I had nothed lost conscious. I ~~~~
also ~~~~ ~~~~ ~~~~ ~~~~ ~~~~ took about
~~~~ left also which ~~which~~ apparrentel
a good ~~~~ a complitly or ~~~~ ~~~~ partially
~~go~~ heal on ~~or~~ execation — for 1/4 – 3 minuts
on excation. Ophthatiomes thiς thi me
to ~~~~ spasms. He should me me it happedamed.

strength and I sank into a depression. At this point, writing a book crossed my mind. Joe and I talked and then recorded some of our conversation. He started getting more and more interested and made plans for me to tape my conversations so that my aphasia could be measured as it cleared up, and also be compared to my previous speech (we had records from our earlier research together). Joe had seen what I had written about the incident and realized better than I that it was almost unintelligible—so taping was essential.

The first attempt at the book.

Several weeks later Jane and I translated it as follows.

Saturday, May 5, 1973   written by Jan
                                              with my collaboration
                                                   June 28, 1973

I have been in good health. Poor exercise, too much smoking. A routine visit to the internist revealed my blood pressure as 180/90. Since this was not dangerous yet, it was decided to do routine tests before going on blood pressure-lowering medication. Nothing showed up on the tests, which took two or three weeks. Some osteophytes in my neck caused some difficulty in turning my head up.

Two or three times during the weeks I had been having these tests, I had lost control of my legs on first arising in the morning. I had not lost consciousness. I had also lost part of my vision in my left eye during these times, and occasionally on exertion for a quarter of a minute to three minutes. The ophthalmologist assured me that this was due to spasms of the retinal vessels. He suggested that I carry nitroglycerine to expand the retinal vessels.

[Next two sentences untranslatable]

It can be seen from the first draft that aside from a paucity of style, the writing tends to be repetitive and telegraphic, the spelling rapidly deteriorates, and I did not catch all of my mistakes. Writing was also unbearably slow.

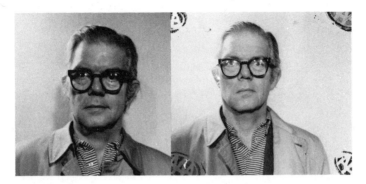

These two passport photos illustrate the paralysis of the right half of my face. The photo on the left was taken six *weeks* after the stroke in anticipation of a vacation abroad. The one on the right was taken six *months* after the stroke, for comparison. I wore the same clothes. The recovery is obvious but not quite complete.

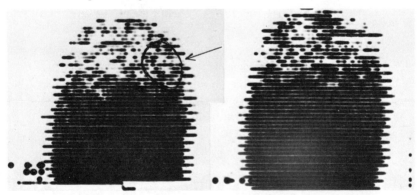

One of the many tests done on me while I was hospitalized was a brain scan. In this test, a short acting, radioactive compound is injected into a vein. This compound is selectively absorbed by certain tissues—one of which is normal brain tis-

sue. Small, evenly spaced x-ray shots are taken on one strip
of film. Damaged brain tissue shows up as a darkish area
(circled and indicated by an arrow) in the left photo of my
brain, taken a few days after the stroke. The recovered scan
on the right was taken three weeks later. As in the usual
x-ray, the negatives are read. For this book positives were
made.

An angiogram, another test, is a method of visualizing
blood vessels by injecting them with compounds that show
on x-ray. A Dynamic scan or scintigram has been called the
poor man's or wise man's angiogram because it gives less information than an angiogram but is also less dangerous. The
same compound used in the brain scan is injected in an arm
vein, and a gamma camera is placed over the neck to measure
how much of the substance is going through each of the two
main arteries that supply the brain. In my case, less (though
still enough) was passing through the left artery. This showed
that there was interference in the blood flow on the left.

One part of the eye exam that I had is called ophthal-
modynamometry. The eye is anesthetized and the pupil is
dilated. A slit lamp is focused on the main branch of the artery in the back of the eye and the operator watches it under
high magnification. A second operator presses an instrument
on the eye which reads the amount of pressure it takes to stop
the blood from flowing through the artery watched by the
first operator.

In my case, shortly after my stroke it took about three-
quarters as much pressure to cut off the blood supply to the
left eye than it did to the right. Though both readings were
within normal limits, they should have been equal. This finding is consistent with the Dynamic scan which showed less
blood flowing through the left neck artery.

An Electroencephalogram (EEG) greatly magnifies and
traces the brain waves (electrical potential). Damaged tissue

yields abnormal tracings as seen above from my brain, approximately three days after my stroke.

Whenever I tell anybody about my stroke the first question is, "In retrospect, could you see it coming?" That's a hard question. Here are the facts.

About two years before the stroke, I had a routine eye ex-

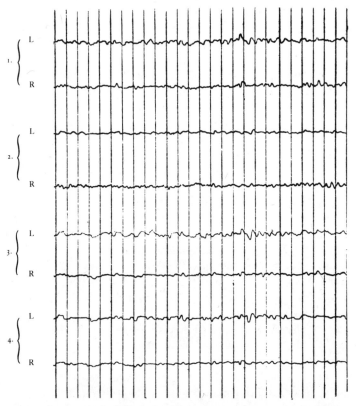

Brain wave record (Electroencephalogram or EEG) taken during Clay's hospitalization from four symmetrical locations on his skull. In each location, the rhythm appears to be slower on the left (L) side of the head than on the right (R). This slowing is most marked in location 3, which was directly over the language areas.

amination. My ophthalmologist, Marvin Gillman, usually recommended only a slight change in glasses, but conscientiously checked lens, retina, etc. The retina is a magnificent device located at the back of the eye. In it you can see a small part of the brain (optic nerve) and a network of the tiniest arteries and veins that the human body possesses.

On this occasion Gillman noticed two or three bubbles on the vessels, rather like a balloon that develops a bump at a thin point as you are blowing it up. In the retinal vessel these bumps are due to back pressure caused by a hardened artery lying across a soft vein. When the artery hardens it is like an iron pipe crossing and pressing down on a rubber hose. The rubber hose constricts, pressure builds up behind it, and sometimes a little bump appears at a weak point. In the same way, the hardened artery (iron pipe) constricts the vein (rubber hose) and a bump or bubble will appear in the vein.

He wanted a retinal specialist to examine me, but neither the doctor I chose nor the one he sent me to found any of the bubbles. Naturally I was a bit suspicious of Gillman's diagnosis. But he found two more bubbles in the next examination and off I went to a specialist again, who took pictures this time, examined them carefully and agreed with Gillman.

The usual cause of these bubbles is arteriosclerosis (hardening of the arteries), often associated with high blood pressure and diabetes, and the specialist gave me four instructions. First, a low animal fat diet (polyunsaturated) since we now know that arteriosclerosis has something to do with cholesterol and a high animal fat diet. I had been following this regime myself with reasonable care for some time, but I suppose I should have started about the time of birth. It takes years of the wrong diet for arteriosclerosis to build up.

The second instruction was to keep my blood thin. One way to accomplish this was to be a blood donor. I didn't pay much attention to this, but I did go to a blood specialist who found nothing wrong. The point in keeping the blood dilute is to reduce clotting possibilities; thick blood tends to clot. Scratch your finger, it bleeds for a few minutes and soon clots; that's good. But a clot in a vessel will clog the vessel; in the brain or heart that's bad. Since I tend to perspire heavily, I was also told to try to avoid perspiring because it further thickens the blood, and to drink lots of water in hot weather. The third instruction was to take nonviolent exercise. I did not follow this conscientiously. The fourth was to see my internist and be checked for diabetes; none was found. Gillman and the specialist agreed that I had mild arteriosclerosis in my eye, which is sometimes connected with heart attacks, sometimes affects the brain, and sometimes less important arteries.

Leland checked the fat in my blood several times but the level was not alarming. About a month before the stroke he noted a rise in my blood pressure to 180 over 90—not a particularly dangerous level, but it had risen. He made some tests to determine if anything unusual had happened. All the tests came out normal as he expected and he then gave me medication to lower the pressure.

I returned to him with new symptoms. On two occasions, when getting out of bed in the morning, I was dizzy, my legs buckled, and my left eye blurred. Once I'd fallen to the floor, and another time caught myself in time on the stair bannister so I didn't lose consciousness. After that I arose more slowly in the morning and sat for a few moments on the edge of the bed before standing up. The condition is called postural hypotension which is something that many people experience—getting dizzy when they get up quickly.

Dr. Leland was quite concerned, however, and said he wanted to refer me to a neurologist who might do brain scans and other tests. This was the first time that the possibility of my own physical disaster seemed real to me. (I could control my overt anxiety but not my gut, and took off for the bathroom.) I asked Leland if he was thinking of brain tumors or other dysfunctions. He said, "Well, we've got to rule them out."

The next step was a thorough examination by the neurologist. This was Zeugma, an excellent doctor with a rather brusque manner but remarkably decent. There was no abnormality and I was to be watched. That was the day before the stroke.

Nothing terribly alarming had occurred to warrant a sense of urgency or any unusual treatment. No one made any further suggestion about the clotting. There are a number of drugs on the market which tend to prevent clotting, but there is no proof that they prevent strokes or heart attacks and there are certain dangers associated with them. Of these drugs, it has recently been learned that aspirin is the safest and easiest to use. I asked Leland about this after the stroke since I didn't remember whether he had prescribed aspirin before. He said, "No, but in retrospect perhaps I should have." As soon as I got to the hospital I was given aspirin rectally in the hope that any clot that formed would not enlarge. As nearly as I can tell from my rapid recovery, this worked out.

To return to the question: could it have been predicted? It was, in a sense, seen as a possibility—but not as a strong enough probability to institute drastic preventive measures. The wisdom of hindsight is always superior.

2

Recovery

I had graduated from hospital to home. Aside from medical checkups the problem was now my own. My body had to regain its functions; I had to work within the limits of fatigue to try to restore my mental and physical self. Moreover, I had to determine what was regainable. That was impossible to know, but I could hope for the best.

Leland and Zuegma decided that I could supervise, determine, and administer my own rehabilitative therapy. This was a good decision. It gave me confidence in my own judgment and kept me from excessive dependency. The specific details emphasized in the story of my recovery are only examples. Other patients would choose different ones.

A description of my home and daily routine during the first weeks may clarify some aspects of what follows.

I live in a private house in Manhattan, the kind of house that is rapidly disappearing from the city. It's narrow and tall; someone described it as a ranch house tipped on edge. It's about sixteen feet wide and four stories high, with two rooms on each floor. There is a small garden in the back. The house allows me to have my office in my home, and avoid the frustrations of New York City. I don't have to travel to work or deal with crowds, buses, taxis, cars and parking problems.

The early days of recovery were devoted to managing my new life, gaining strength, and testing my functioning. My "stroke personality"—the good, undemanding patient—still dominated.

When I arrived home from the hospital I was allowed to go downstairs once a day. At first my breakfast was brought to me in bed on the third floor. Blood circulation tends to be sluggish after a long sleep, and I presume that is why my mornings were so difficult. For many months it took me about two hours to wake up and move around slowly until I felt "normal." For many months Jane couldn't understand anything I said during the first hour. This condition gradually improved, but for at least a year Jane brought me coffee in bed to help me wake up.

After a few days I had a table set up in my study, also on the third floor. I had breakfast there and spent the rest of the morning in the garden. After lunch I returned to the third floor for the rest of the day, which included dinner with Jane and Jim. They were always warm, attentive, perceptive, and sympathetic.

Jane comments: In the first few weeks I described our house as "all stairs." Clay not only needed meals brought to him, but countless other items he wanted to use, look at, and so forth. He was not aware of how Jim and I developed our leg muscles in fetching and carrying. When he was on the third floor I would say, "I am going downstairs. Is there anything you want?" No, he couldn't think of a thing. When I returned he remembered something, but only one thing at a time. There are advantages to a home with stairs, but not with a stroke victim in the family.

I suffered from the physical effects of not using my legs. I would pace the floor in the evening; back and forth from the bedroom, down the hall to my study, around a circle and back again, like a caged animal. My legs needed to move. (It wasn't until later that I began to feel the pain and aching from trying to exercise them back into shape.)

Muscles have one function; contraction, and its corollary, relaxation, in order to produce movement. When this doesn't occur, the muscles start to atrophy. But I had to move my legs slowly, particularly on the stairs, in order to avoid strain and undue fatigue. Since I was in no rush to go anywhere this made little difference, and since I misjudged the height of the steps I had to climb even more carefully to avoid tripping.

My family and friends were my gophers ("gophers" go for things). I wanted to do some necessary house repairs and work on my amateur sculpture, but shortly discovered that I had neither the physical nor mental ability to do much. Sculpture requires concentration over a period of several hours and I was just not up to it. A repair also, even a small one, demands a steady hand and I didn't have it. For instance, I was shocked to discover that after I had taken something apart I couldn't find the screws that needed to be replaced. I'm not sure, but I think I was merely repairing an appliance plug. So those activities were out and I was left with passive ways to spend time.

Jim writes: One of the hardest aspects of the stroke for me to accept was that Dad, who was always a very dynamic, energetic, and physically strong person and a model for me as I was growing up, had been weakened physically. His memory had also been affected. My model during adolescence suddenly was changed and weakened. And this just at the point when I was excelling, so an exchange of an "energy package" seemed to take place. (I find it difficult to know that Dad is reading this.) I have, since the stroke occurred, felt a loss—not just personally or to my father—but also on principle, as when one reads in the newspaper of a great luxury liner burning.

The Watergate hearings were just beginning and they were a lifesaver. I was glued to the set—whether in the garden or upstairs in my study. It was sometimes hard for me to tell one witness from another and to remember names, but it amused me to think that if I had been one of those liars I would have blessed the memory loss and difficulty in speaking that the aphasia offered me.

The weekends, and other times when there was no Watergate, were a problem. I learned a bit about daytime television. "Sesame Street" was the most enjoyable, probably because it was new to me. Much daytime TV was ghastly but I enjoyed some old movies.

Jane brought me the kind of novels I used to read, and though I could read fairly well, I found them too difficult. Too many characters confused me, so she found some very simple-minded mysteries that had only a few characters. Although my reading and ability to concentrate improved, I still found sentences that were difficult. For example, this sentence was confusing: "But this could be less than a hardship . . ." This conveyed nothing at all to me until I figured out that "less" was the qualification of "hardship" and therefore meant "reasonably easy." That took five to ten minutes.

My other activity was to handicap the horse races and sometimes discuss them with my friend, Jeff Newman, who then made the bets for me. Each evening the gophers went out to get me the next day's Racing Form.

Jane adds: Clay always enjoyed horse racing. During his early recovery, he labored over the racing forms and then made small bets which provided some excitement—awaiting the results at the end of each day. He didn't win often, but he felt it was necessary to back up his judgment with a small wager as an expression of confidence. However, the real problem was in the addition and subtraction in the handicapping.

Jim spent a lot of time with me and did the things I needed done. My instructions were vague: "Put the thing over on the thing—you know, the thing down there." He had been living home all year, partly to save money to outfit his thirty-five-foot yacht. He had originally planned to sail it to Cape Cod in the beginning of May. He delayed leaving for weeks, but his job wouldn't wait and we convinced him to go. It is difficult for parents to see their youngsters take off, and though sad, we were pleased at his competence and independence.

The following is an excerpt from Jim's log, written on his trip alone to the Cape.

I find myself feeling, aside from occasional intense pangs of loneliness, great remorse for Mom and Dad. I have treated them well (and vice versa), but nevertheless I cannot help but feel I have abandoned them during a time of great need. My reason and rationalization of having to live my own life and get to Provincetown only goes so far. Even though it is true, it does not excuse me from some degree of neglect. Mom said (the night before I left New York City) that Dad felt *bereft*. I'm sure he does. I see him as a great, resourceful, and self-sufficient man (what I'm trying to become) suddenly crippled (if that is not too strong a word) or disabled, and unable to use all his talents. Not only did he need me to do jobs around the house, but more importantly, he could take pride in seeing an "image of himself" —something that for the most part he molded and influenced—perform well. My presence, my energy shared with him, helped restore him a little to that level he once had. I may very well be projecting, but if I were in his situation, I would be feeling that way.

It is amazing to me how the feelings of remorse and loneliness are always with me at sea. . . .

Friends were remarkably kind. They had come to the hospital to keep Jane company, taking her out for lunch and dinner. (Jane said later that the most exhausting part of my illness for her were all the friends. While I was in the hospital, she and Jim spent hours in the morning and evenings talking to well-wishers on the phone. However, it is gratifying to know that so many people care.)

When I was home, friends phoned and came to visit, and while all of this was somewhat strenuous, they recognized that I tired easily. I took full advantage of this and cut any visits short when fatigue set in. Jane allowed only one or two people to visit at a time because I became confused when several people talked, and a room full of noise was intolerable.

Two examples of exceptional thoughtfulness stand out. One couple arranged to come on an evening when I felt up to it, bringing my favorite lobster salad which we all ate on my study table. It was a particularly thoughtful thing to do since Jane couldn't invite dinner guests in addition to working and doing all the chores for me.

The other example occurred when I was allowed out of the house several weeks later. Some friends called to say, "If Clay wants to go out for dinner we would like to take you both out, as part of his getting back into the swing of things." I would not have thought of doing this for someone in my position and the idea both terrified and delighted me.

Jane suggested we go to a small restaurant early in the evening to avoid crowds and noise. I still did not have complete control of my mouth, and Jane occasionally gave me signals. When she put her hand to her lip I used the napkin. I could then eat with reasonable assurance that I was not being too slobbery. It all went off well and I was enormously reassured; I could manage a meal in public.

Getting back into a social scene was a boost to my self-esteem and relieved boredom, but it was easy to overtax myself.

About two weeks after I was allowed to leave the house I insisted that we make our annual outing with Jeff and Killy Newman to the Belmont Stakes—the big race of the year in New York. We had tickets, Secretariat was running, and I was determined to go. Jane and the Newmans were concerned about the strain on me so I agreed to arrive only in time to see the Belmont and one or two other races. I stayed in my seat quietly, but had to stand up and holler when my horse came in. It was a good day. Secretariat set a record, winning by thirty-one lengths. I remember feeling I was thirty-one lengths ahead. In this mood I agreed that we all go out for dinner after the races. Dinner was delightful, but when I got home the fatigue was exceptional and I succumbed to depression and self-pity. I recall lying down on the bed and asking Jane to sit beside me. I wept and said I was shot, and would never be myself again. Later, the mood passed.

I was first allowed out of the house on May 24, exactly one month after my stroke. It was a great day. Leland called to tell me that my brain scan was clear, and that I could go out and start having some more exercise—"mild and careful." I rushed to call Jane at her office. She mentioned that it was cloudy out but I thought it looked wonderful. I went for a short walk and was ecstatic. Being turned loose meant many things. It was spring; I could get around, see people on the streets, and change my routine.

I could now also overlook Leland's last injunction to me in the hospital about sex. When Johnny and I tried to see the naked lady across from the hospital, it was not for my sexual enjoyment. I have voyeuristic tendencies but they weren't active then. Nor did I have sex on my mind except to wonder when the desire would return. One morning, however, about three weeks poststroke, I woke up with an erection and it was a pleasant sensation. Life was coming back to me. So very shortly after I was cleared by the latest brain scan, we decided it was time for action. I think we were both nervous but all went well and afterward Jane asked me how I felt. Since the question could have had two meanings, I replied "Good," asked her the same question and got the same reply. I think that aside from the greater fatigue and the ordinary slowing down that comes with age in men, I am sexually about where I was before the stroke.

I have heard it said that following a stroke, sex is finished. I want to clear up that misapprehension now. It is true, of course, the certain physical difficulties such as hand or leg paralysis might alter some sexual athletics. But physical difficulties do not alter orgasmic potential. What may happen, and frequently does, is that the emotional depression following a stroke (and most chronic diseases) severely limits sexual as well as any other interest. But this is not a physical disability, and if the emotional depression can be overcome, sexuality can rapidly return to normal and even help alleviate the depression.

One of the first things I did when I was turned loose was to go to an art store and find one of the lightweight stools on which art students sit when sketching in a gallery. New York City has few public benches. I carried the stool with me for about a month so if I got tired I could sit down wherever I was. Age fifty is not the same as twenty; one recovers much more slowly from illness and its attendant inactivity. I suffered leg cramps when I was tottering around town. This was tolerable although as I exercised harder the cramps increased. The freedom to go out was enhanced by the freedom of rest wherever I was on my stool.

A cane followed the stool. This served a dual function: I could lean on it when I had to, but more importantly, it made me look like a cripple. Sometimes I used it a bit more ostentatiously than necessary, because people make room for cripples and I was, in fact, afraid of crowds. I didn't want to be hit and toppled over. My strength and coordination were poor and I was fearful that a blow to my head or neck might knock another plaque loose from an artery. Fear prompted me to improve my manners on the street; when people were rude (in typical big city ways) I didn't holler back or shout imprecations. I merely said, "Excuse me."

As I moved around more, I learned to discard my casual approach to other dangers, such as stairs and street crossings. I learned to hold on to bannisters and wait for street lights to change. I took other precautions such as carrying a flashlight in the dark, particularly when groping my way to the bathroom. Baths replaced showers until I felt surer of not slipping on the porcelain floor.

My clumsiness was particularly noticeable in the house where I repeatedly bumped into table legs. An important lesson learned was not to go barefoot—kicking a table leg hurts and one may slip. Not infrequently, I kicked Jane's rocking chair. When I mentioned this to her, she said, "You always did that. The difference is you now say 'Excuse me.'" Maybe she's right.

My coordination problems extended beyond clumsiness. My hands and arms were affected, as well as my voice, speech, and mouth muscles.

I had been home about two weeks when I had to write some checks. I spent fifteen or twenty minutes practicing my signature with Jane's help until she decided it was legible. Writing checks was only one of countless examples of minor changes in lifestyle to adapt to physical limitations. Although I could sign my name, Jane had to fill in the rest of the check. She kept forgetting, and often signed her own name on my bank account.

Seven months poststroke I could write about a page, but spelling was difficult. At first I could not even copy a word accurately. Nor could I write when anyone else was talking. I worked like a third-grader who sticks out his tongue and pushes with his left hand while writing with his right, because after about two hundred words my arms felt as if they were about to fall off. I must have been pushing very hard with both arms.

Jane, who has been a college teacher all of her adult life, has learned to read almost any kind of handwriting. As soon as I could write at all, I would write down a thought—("Ask Joe about Sam," "Send someone to get paper," and the like. Later Jane would read these and translate them into English because I was usually unable to read my scribbles. This improved with time, and we preserved some of these notes. One word we puzzled over for a long time looked like "know-horry." It is still a mystery, although Jane now thinks it may have meant "no hurry"; however we no longer have the context in which it was written.

I have a fine tremor in my right hand, more than in the left. When Joe and I wanted to test and compare the progress in my coordination and the difference between fine movements in each hand, we searched for some common, everyday activity which would be easily observable and useful for comparisons. Typing would have been ideal, but I can't type. With most activities one uses the preferred hand if it is convenient. We finally hit on a good comparison. There is only one way to button a shirt sleeve—with the opposite hand—and most people learn to be ambidextrous in this task. A year after the stroke I still fumbled with my right hand when buttoning my left sleeve. I am not sure how much of my continued fumbling is due to a lack of feeling in my fingers, and how much is the failure to make fine movements—perhaps it is a bit of both.

When Joe suggested that I dictate and tape-record my notes for this book, he also wanted a running record of my speech and language improvement. We decided that I should recite the alphabet, as a standard task which could be compared day by day. We felt I should also tape some simple sentences so I took to reading the "Quotation of the Day," from *The New*

York Times which was interesting. Of course, these were not comparable in terms of vocabulary and grammatical complexity. Perhaps there are more uniform reading tests but we didn't know of them. Reading the same sentence every day would have been of less value because of the improvement due to sheer practice—rather than brain recovery. An example from a "Quotation of the Day," as dictated by me, follows.

The President is very concerned at having persevered to . . . long years, since Congress . . . negotiations . . . severely undermines prospects for success.

The actual quotation was:

The President is very concerned that having persevered to success these long years, the Congress has, on the eve of negotiations to achieve compliance with that settlement, taken action that could severely undermine prospects for success.[1]

I had a hard time reading that into the dictating machine, and the typist had an even harder time transcribing it. It was very hard for me to understand what Nixon was saying, but as I also dictated at the time, "Nixonese is always hard to understand." I did better with other quotes.

My voice had also changed. A friend told me that I spoke like Marlon Brando. I knew I mumbled, but I had also lost a certain sonorousness. The voice quality came back in about four months but I still mumble when I'm tired. And I am tired of being tired.

Jane writes: When Clay could talk again in the hospital, he not only mumbled; his voice was very thick and often so unintelligible that we had to continue playing charades for me to understand certain things he was saying. When one of his patients told me on the phone how distressed she felt about his stroke, I suggested she phone Clay,

1. Statement on Indochina by President Nixon; "Quotation of the Day" May 17, 1973, *The New York Times.*

but warned her that his voice was thick—he sounded drunk. People couldn't recognize his voice on the phone.

I got used to the stroke voice and really didn't notice the gradual improvement (one doesn't when you're that close every day—it takes others to point out improvements). But there actually was huge improvement which was brought home several months later. I was upstairs working at my desk and Clay was two flights below, in his office. I suddenly heard that ghastly voice—that early stroke voice—and went running downstairs in a panic, thinking that he'd had another stroke. He was listening to a replay of an early tape he'd made.

There are certain words that remain difficult for me to pronounce. There is more about this in a later chapter, but it might be worthwhile here to say something about this difficulty in my daily life. An insurance man came around to see if I was really disabled. I spoke about my disability "polithy," a "th" sound replacing the "c." I think this has to do with the position of the tongue between the two vowels. The aphasic learns certain strategies for dealing with such things. One strategy was to pause between the two words, "disability" and "policy." A second more useful strategy for me was to change the second word and just say "disability insurance," which came quite easily. Another word which was a tongue twister was "witchcraft." When it once came up in a conversation, I said it rapidly and it turned out to be "whichcrap." That turned out to be rather funny since that is what I think of witchcraft. If it now comes up in a conversation I leave it that way.

One last point about my voice. I'm not much of a singer but I can carry a tune. I found early on that I could sing a song I knew well (mostly "la de da" because I never did know all the words) much better than I could speak. Something about the music carries one along. Stutterers have long known this. Singing familiar songs is easer for an aphasic than talking.

Some of the problems I experienced in being in touch with the world again involved numbness in my face, a diminished sense of taste, and the strain of conflicting voices which made

me particularly sensitive to interruption. Others noticed my
unawareness of errors I made in speaking and in writing, and
Joe explains this in a later chapter.

In describing numbness I have previously used the analogy
of dental anesthesia, but it is not really like that. In my experience, when I had dental anesthesia I sometimes bit my
tongue or cheek and they felt thick and insensitive. But with
anesthesia I also could not feel the dentist's drill. This type of
numbness is due to a partial loss of feeling. However, since
some feeling remains, the subjective effect is that of a *different*
sensation rather than an *absence* of sensation. For example, a
pin stuck simultaneously on each side of my face was not as
sharp on the right side as the left, but I could still feel it.
Food got stuck in my mouth on the right side without my noticing it. At one time, when I was eating some cherries during the summer, putting three or four at a time into my
mouth as I have done since childhood, I didn't spit out all the
pits; a few minutes later I found one or two pits in the corner
of my right cheek. My lip still sags on the right side a little
and small amounts of drooling can occur which I don't notice.
(I've gotten into the habit of inconspicuously wiping my
mouth frequently.)

The numbness extends beyond my face. I will frequently
turn over two pages of a book at one time with my right
fingers. At first I thought this was accidental because the
books were new, but when it kept happening with old books
I realized that I lacked sensitivity in the right hand.

Probably most distressing was the difficulty in dealing with
conflicting voices and sounds. I could only cope with one
thought, one sound, and one situation at a time. Awareness
can at times be general; when you are not concentrating intensely on one thing, you can be aware of several things simultaneously. Ordinarily, you can converse while crossing
the street and watching traffic. You can watch TV and do
some handiwork. You can listen to someone talk, and take
notes. After the stroke I could receive only one input at a
time; more than that was chaos. Although Jane limited visitors to one or two at a time, unexpected visitors sometimes

arrived. I'm afraid I was quite rude then because I became tense and confused and shut people off. If I was talking, any interruption made me lose my train of throught. The same happened with my own interruptions. When struggling to find the right word I would forget what I was trying to say.

We had planned a trip to Scandinavia many months prior to the stroke and I was determined to go. When Zeugma finally agreed and told me to enjoy myself, I was exuberant, but then problems arose.

I left to meet Sidney for lunch, and on my way stopped at a bank to get travelers checks for the trip. I had to fill out a brief form, sign my name on the checks fifteen times, and write a check for the total sum. By the time I was through, I found that for the first time my right leg was dragging and my mind was unclear. I got to Sidney's office, but he had to put me in a taxi and send me home. I had had difficulties with strength and coordination (writing my name so often, leg muscles); with concentration (handling so many pieces of paper, a clouded mind); with language (counting the number of checks and writing a total amount); and with emotions (unrealistic expectations of myself and psychological depression following the physical exhaustion).

It turned out that one of the great advantages of going to Scandinavia that summer was that there was virtually no pressure on me to manage customary social situations. I received no phone calls. Since I could scarcely use my own language, there was no point in trying to learn Norwegian or Danish. All I had to learn was the equivalent of "excuse me" for occasions when I bumped into people. Jane and I were alone most of the time and I had her undivided attention.

It has been said, and I think with some truth, that I am stubborn. While I was still in the hospital Jane suggested we postpone our trip, but I was determined to go. It seemed an important part of my recovery to carry through the plans we had made. A fair amount of the trip was boring since I suffered the usual fatigue, but I would have been bored some of the time anywhere that summer.

Packing for the trip was tense. Although Jane did most of

it for me, I thought I could manage certain common items such as socks, underwear, and toilet articles, but it became a hassle for me. It wouldn't have mattered if I forgot some items because we could have bought them overseas. I made lists only Jane could read, and she would then rewrite them for my use. I would make piles for packing and get more and more tense. As I was packing I heard myself saying aloud, "Easy, take it easy, no rush, take it easy, no rush, don't forget raincoat, all right, take it easy."

Making travel arrangements was hopeless for me and I made no attempt to cope with them. Jane attended to details, asked questions, and handled situations that at the time seemed too complex for me. Since I'd grown up in middle-class America, I was used to taking care of "masculine" details. I signed into hotels, picked up the bags, gave taxi directions, and ordered in restaurants. I couldn't do any of these things now and Jane managed marvelously. This reversal of roles was not too hard on me. I had by this time learned some of my limitations, and fortunately I had someone to depend upon. I even got to enjoy this passive role in some ways—as I had in the early hospital days.

Jane adds: It wasn't too hard on me either, but I looked forward to the time Clay would be able to do the managing again. It wasn't the physical exertion I minded as much as the loss of my female enjoyment of being "taken care of."

When there were no distractions, I enjoyed many of our sightseeing trips intensely. One cold foggy day, sailing on the Norwegian fiords, I was the only person to spend the entire trip outdoors on the ferry deck. It was an unforgettable experience which I concentrated on and savored to the fullest. I remembered my father's descriptions of his Scandinavian childhood. In the elegant prose of the late John McNulty I felt that I was "back where I had never been."

However, I wasn't always so full of equanimity. One rainy day in Denmark we had trouble finding a place to eat and were tired and irritable when we finally found a cafeteria.

Jane took the tray, which wasn't big enough for all we selected, and I asked her to rearrange the plates. She didn't hear me so I took the tray and tried to put another cup of coffee on it. I was carrying my cane and bumped it into the man behind me. Finally, I got it all together, and then had to pay for the food at the end of the cafeteria line. This meant I had to do the calculations in Danish kroners. I became intensely confused, and must have been shouting at Jane which embarrassed her. The multiplicity of events coming all at once, and my inability to cope, hit me. I was badly shaken and sat down in a chair. My hands trembled as I rubbed my aching legs.

That night I had a nightmare: Jane and I were in a car in a foreign place I had never seen, with lots of water and many houses. I got angry at her, left, and walked back to where I had come from—where I knew she could find me. It wasn't too far away and I was rushing along. There was no pain or shortness of breath—I was in my prestroke state. I passed a number of places which looked quite nice; some had ponds filled with fish. Then Jane appeared in the background two or three times, and I was lost in a house and had a hard time getting out. It was not my house and I didn't want the people who lived there to see me. I woke up.

Without going into all the possible meanings of this dream, I think it was a dramatic description of my dependency on her, my difficulty in taking a passive role, and how lost I was without her. When I dictated the following note in Denmark, full of self-pity, I said, "I can't even throw a fit properly." Of course I had had a hell of a fit in the cafeteria. I think my denial of this meant that the fit was ineffective or even harmful.

A few days after the cafeteria panic we went to Tivoli Gardens in Copenhagen. We had dinner and walked about. It's a lovely place and the people were nice. Areas in the gardens were like a carnival—crowded and noisy—but curiously that didn't bother me. We played slot machines, bingo (in Danish), and several spinning wheel games of chance. I dropped my cane several times and was very excited, but it was all fun. It was entirely different from the cafeteria and much more hectic. I think the difference was in my self-consciousness. In the cafeteria my gaucheness and inadequacy bothered me. When I was having fun I forgot about myself.

The same ability to manage crowds and stimulating events was evident when we went to the horse races in Denmark. While very different from an American track, a similar excitement pervaded the crowd. Although Jane had to find out how to make the bets and read the program, for some reason I wasn't concerned about coping and simply enjoyed life. The noise around me became a distant murmur.

Jane says I try to hog attention when I'm in a group. This is true at times when I'm prone to making wisecracks and irrelevancies. Although this is an extension of my prestroke personality, it is not just a matter of getting attention. By cutting off other people I can lessen the distraction of multiple voices. Of course, it can be disruptive and sometimes I get hell for it.

My memory after the stroke was bad, but I was also easily intimidated. For example, I went to see Sidney at his office, which I rarely do. His office is in a large midtown building which has an east and west side. There is a directory on the wall and each office has an E or W after the office number. An attendant told me Sid's office was on the twenty-fourth floor in the west building. I really thought it was east, but I followed his directions and was totally confused by my lack of familiarity with the floor when I got there. I went downstairs again and looked on the board myself and saw that I had been right; it was on the east side. By then I was more confused. Someone else asked me where I wanted to go and I said "fourteenth floor." When I calmed down I pushed the twenty-fourth floor button. This kind of incident became common, but I'm not sure it's loss of memory. When you don't trust yourself you're easily intimidated by people who seem positive, and when they are wrong the confusion increases.

The most serious consequences of my stroke were due to aphasia; that is, my difficulty reading in the hospital, the problem of understanding complex plots in novels or in the

Watergate hearings, the problem of conflicting voices, finding the right words, and writing difficulties.

The most striking demonstration of aphasia was in the simplest tasks—reciting the alphabet or counting. When Zeugma asked me to say the alphabet, the day before I left the hospital, I did it very slowly. I stumbled somewhere around the middle, but was able to finish correctly. The middle letters continued to be difficult to dictate. I could have cheated by just reading off a phone dial but I was much more interested in the process than in fooling anyone. I had a persistent problem with the letter "U," either dropping it or putting it in twice. Later someone asked me why I always counted on my knuckles while reciting the alphabet. The reason was to know if I ended up with 26 letters; it was helpful even when I was correct, which I found on reading the tape transcription I sometimes was. In about four months I managed the alphabet without much difficulty and with my usual rapidity. However, even though I was able to recite it sequentially, I had trouble using it.

Who uses the alphabet consciously after second grade? It's only necessary when you are looking up a word in a telephone book, dictionary, or card catalogue. If a word begins with the letter "S," do you start with "A?" Of course not. Imagine you are looking for the letter which follows "S" in the word, perhaps a "P." In order to find "SP" I had to start much further back with "SL, SM, SN, SO," and finally "SP." This is both difficult and slow. I can do it now but it does not come with ease.

Two months after the stroke I wanted to get a new head for my electric razor. I spent twenty minutes with the Yellow Pages and finally, in a sweat, asked Jane to look up the store. I was within three pages but couldn't find it. After I had purchased the razor head, I couldn't install it because the directions were mildly complex. I was directed to: "Remove the head, first pushing the blades to the down position and to the left, and insert new blades from the right, keeping them in the proper numerical order." Clearly this was not written with the aphasic in mind.

Spelling was another problem. First I had to ask for simple words and later more complicated ones. I learned to divide words into syllables. Once I wanted to find "monkey" in the dictionary. Expecting no trouble, I found "M," then "MO" and tried for "MOK." After several minutes of running my hand up and down the page, I printed out "MONKEY," saw my error and found the word. I could spell it correctly in my head, but I couldn't retain it long enough while using the dictionary.

When Joe and I first started recording my daily notes, he suggested that I try numbers—counting and calculations. Doing numbers turned out to be quite easy and practice helped, but I had problems with double digits. One of my first exercises came out like this: "1, 2, 3, 4, 5, 6, 7, 8, 9 (long pause), 9, (long pause), *one oh.*" I simply could not say ten. Naturally I practiced saying "ten." Then I progressed to counting 10, 11, 12 . . . which went along pretty well, followed by 10, 20, 30, 40, etc.

When I was a psychiatric resident we had a test in which people were asked to start 100 and subtract serial 7s; that is, 100, 93, 86, 79, 72, 65, 58, 51, 44, 37, 30, 23, 16, 9, 2. This is to see if one can concentrate reasonably well, keep track of a result, and use it again in an arithmetic operation. This is the quote from the tape: "100, 97, let's start again. 93, 96, 79, 79, 72, 33, (long pause), 72, (long pause), 30, ah, ah, 65, 80, ah. I'm stopping that now; my brain is getting very tired." That scared me so much that I didn't try it again for another month. I did much better the next time although I was not perfect. (Seven months later I got to 50 and knew I had made a mistake. The only zero number you reach in the series is 30.)

In using numbers, I mixed up the meaning of figures that had several zeros. I would quite often shock Jane with the figures I quoted. If I cashed a check I would tell her it was for $5,000 instead of $500, and once I told her we had $2 million in the bank instead of $2,000.

Despite my confusion, when Jane was filling out a form for me shortly after I left the hospital and asked if I knew my social security number, I reeled off the nine numbers correctly with no hesitation. Big Brother must have imprinted them on my brain in 1935. Yet, I could scarcely dial a phone with the number right in front of me.

The dates on my dictated recordings were a mess. I tried to do them by memory and then check a calendar for accuracy, but found that the years as well as the months were wrong, although the days were easier. For a long time I reported the year "1973" as "1972," and sometimes as "1937" or "1927." The months were even worse. I could not remember that my stroke occurred on April 24 (and seven months later as I wrote this, I dictated April 21); the most frequent month I used for dates was March, the one prior to the stroke.

The following is a psychological explanation of the problem of dates, and like all psychological formulations it is hypothetical.

Some confusion about dates is normal. Most people automatically date checks with last year's date after New Year's Day, and it may even take a few months until the new year is automatic. My reverting to 1972 in April, 1973 was an exaggeration of a normal experience.

Getting stuck on the month of March, the month *prior* to the stroke, is something else. In traumatic brain injuries, such as a physical blow to the head, there is often an amnesia for the event itself as well as some time prior to the accident. For example, a fighter who has been knocked out may not remember the fight when he comes to, and may even think it is the day before the fight. This amnesia disappears as he recovers from the concussion, and soon he remembers the beginning of the fight, but perhaps not the round in which he was knocked out. Eventually, even that may come back. Rarely can he remember anything from the precise period of unconsciousness. Amnesia, therefore, tends to start before the event and then to shrink during recovery.

The odd thing in my case is that I was never unconscious. I have a clear memory of the moment of the stroke, as well as the events preceding and following it; I am absolutely sure of this. As far as remembering the exact date is concerned, I behaved as though I was knocked unconscious sometime in April, 1973 and was stuck back in March 1973 or even March, 1972. Happily, the rest of my memory didn't show this pattern and I always knew the night of the stroke had been a Tuesday. Of course, I taught on Tuesday nights so it was not a routine day.

The mistake I made in dictating April 21 instead of April 24, though I "knew" the correct date by the time of the dictation, might be a result of aphasic speech disturbance rather than memory loss. The words "first" and "fourth" have the same initial consonant. The aphasic may remember correctly and intend to say one thing, but it may come out differently. If, in addition, he doesn't register the error, he assumes he's said what he intended and proceeds. The principle illustrated by the error may be semantic similarity (use of a wrong but related word) or phonetic similarity, or both (as in the case of "21st" for 24th.")

My ability to handle numerical data definitely improved by the time we were in Scandinavia (three months after the stroke). Many travelers have problems with monetary exchange, and we wanted, like any foreigners, to know what the local money meant in United States dollars. Scandinavian kroner was roughly equal to 20 cents in American money. It's an easy system—just divide 5 into almost anything to get the dollar equivalent. I could not do this however. I could divide 5 into 500, but 5 into 745 was beyond me. Could the computation strategy be simplified? I figured out the algebra of this easily: with a large figure like 7255, drop the final digit and multiply by 2. (Dividing by 10 and multiplying by 2 is the same as dividing by 5.) I could do the algebra but I could not multiply by 2! I think I figured out the equation faster than Jane and she has a good mathematical mind. I may have had more motivation. Needless to say, she paid hotel, restaurant, and other bills.

Motivation, incidentally, is essential to all phases of recovery, from the simplest tasks to writing this book, as well as for all diagnostic testing. My motivation was so great that after I was told to walk as much as possible for exercise I became a "gopher" myself, finding small items needed for the household. The walk then had a goal. (I have heard of a heart attack patient who did comparison shopping in markets until his wife complained about all the ketchup he bought.)

One of my first shopping expeditions was to a houseware store for an electric plug, but I couldn't think of the name "electric plug" and it took me a while to get the message across. Naturally, I was humiliated and frustrated. I am one of those persons who is rather easily brought to tears, usually by music, a poem, or a sensitive subject. This doesn't bother me, in fact it is relieving. I was close to tears at the store, however, and let them out to Jane at home. But I was learning day by day the frustrations of a body and mind I could not command. Too many new situations had to be met and handled.

The aphasia resulted in another difficult situation. Although I had insisted that we go to Scandinavia, Jane might have talked me out of it if we could have anticipated the trouble we had with our car, a stick shift Volkswagen. Jane had always driven an automatic shift so she took a few lessons before we left New York. Although I could drive for short periods, she had to do most of it. Every time she had to think of something besides the clutch, she stalled. On every trip tension was rife, but Copenhagen survived.

My job was navigation. I'm a good map reader, having learned very well during World War II (after I misread a map and came face to face with a German gun). Copenhagen is a marvelous city but it seemed as if the city planners had dumped a can of worms and traced the streets around them. Then, having a sense of history, they named the streets after historical figures. With so many great names to honor they often named every block or two after a different person. Therefore, at some intersections the street had a different name in each direction. For instance, Hans Christian Anderson Street turns into Dag Hammarskjöld Street.

I would look at the maps and ascertain that a right turn was in order and would then say, "Turn left." Jane followed my instructions. "I said left." Jane: "I turned left." Clay: "No, I

said left." Jane: "It is left." Then the car stalled. I had not
heard myself say "left" when I meant "right." These exercises
were carried out with a maximum of noise until I figured out
that I *knew* what direction I meant but couldn't be relied on
to *name* the correct direction. We solved the problem by my
sticking my hand in front of her nose to point left or right.

I did better with my visual memory. If I had been some-
place before, I was good at finding it again. I've since learned
that it is the right half of the brain (my healthy side) which
controls that function.

There were numerous other aphasic and memory problems. Everyone tells some stories repeatedly, but within fifteen minutes I repeated three stories that Jane had already
just heard—from me. That's a little too much, even for a
raconteur! When I became irritated with her for telling me,
she reminded me that it probably was a favor to do so. I
agreed, but it was not easy. My self-image is surely not that
of a bore.

The above experiences have not brought me humility but
they have at least taught me to control my temper. I have lost
some confidence, but this is not the whole basis of control. I
hope that I have developed a true regard for, or at least patience with, other people. "Excuse me" is becoming a habit
and I hope it continues to be one because it seems to make
other people feel better and therefore behave better towards
me. When tensions build up and the blow-up comes, it can
be expressed as sarcasm, a raised voice, or simply leaving the
room and trying to calm down. The suppressed annoyance,
anger, whatever, remains and sometimes erupts—usually toward the one who is with me most—Jane.

In the first dream I remembered, about three weeks after
the stroke, I was looking at the television movie listings in the
newspaper and noticed a film named "Coma." The capsule
comment following the listing said "Inhuman out there." Although I had not had a coma, nor been aware up to this point
of anxiety, perhaps the anxiety came out in my sleep, and
also in fantasies.

A few months later I remembered a shoemaker I had

known as a young man. He put tacks in his mouth, spat them out and pounded them into the shoe very dexterously. My fantasy was of his having a stroke and swallowing the tacks— my first stroke symptom was choking.

Anxiety is a natural response to catastrophic illness. It is an uncomfortable feeling which everyone experiences when integrity is threatened, and we acquire a host of ways to avoid the feeling. Perhaps my "stroke personality" in the early days of illness was one such mechanism. Although the defenses against anxiety usually work quite well to help us function from day to day, the problem is still there and may appear in other ways, such as in dreams.

I don't think I am especially vain but I am sometimes arrogant. I try to focus this into an ambition towards excellence in my work, tempered with the knowledge that, at best, my guesses can only be shrewd and not perfect. This, accompanied by a knowledge of the failures, throughout history, of people who thought they were right and were proven wrong, has served me fairly well. I have learned over the years to say, "I don't know." Aphasia, and the physical disabilities accompanying a stroke, even a mild one such as mine, deflects the tendency toward arrogance, but doesn't completely abolish it. If one were to have foreknowledge of a stroke, I suppose humility would be a better personality characteristic to cultivate.

My arrogance was being chipped away by repeated instances of not knowing, not remembering, and being proven wrong. An increase in humility was illustrated to me by my dream of staples being stuck in my hands and feet. I had never thought of myself as being, in any fashion, "Christlike," but of course these were staples and not nails. The point was how I felt about myself at the time. I felt scarcely worth bothering about, and staples would do instead of nails. I suppose the reason why I had these things stuck in me was because I was very depressed at the time of the dream.

Depression is the most difficult problem. Jane reports that

most people who inquired about me once they knew I was recovering, asked "How are his spirits?" The honest answer is up and down.

The depression I refer to comes from a sense of loss of a cherished possession. It may be the death of a loved one, an object stolen, or a fantasy dispelled—such as not getting a job one wanted, a date, or a publisher for a book. In my case the loss was a significant part of my body's ability to function.

The symptoms of depression are many. The face droops, the body slumps and moves slowly, appetite diminishes (or sometimes increases to combat depression), and mental processes slow down. Sometimes physical activity of a nonproductive type appears, such as drumming fingers or pacing the floor. Anger may be prominent, or self-pity. Whining and placing blame are probably the least pleasant for others to hear as well as for one's self.

Jane: When Clay started complaining regularly when I returned home from work, I told him I realized what a "fishwife" is. It has nothing to do with gender. It's a syndrome of the person left alone at home, with not enough to do, and feeling depressed. After that, Clay stopped being a "fishperson" much of the time.

The worst outcome of depression is usually considered to be suicide. That, at least, requires an active decision. Perhaps apathy is even worse.

The depressive needs companionship, but his behavior drives people away. There are a number of reasons for this, but it is mostly because he or she is a self-preoccupied bore, or because he brings out the depressive potential in all of us. Psychiatrists generally agree that they could not cope with talking to one depressive patient after another all day; one's own depressive potential becomes activated. One depression is much the same as the next. You feel awful, you don't see how it's going to get better, and nobody wants to listen to a lot of that.

We say the wrong things to depressives: "Cheer up"; "It can't be that bad"; all of which drives them deeper into their depression. The message they detect is: "I don't want to hear about it," or "I don't understand you."

Jane: Since the stroke, I've learned from Clay that when he is feeling depressed there is no point in discussing it with him. Nothing I can say will make him feel better. Besides, I figure he has something legitimate to feel depressed about.

Since depression is a sense of loss, I'm mostly set off by some disappointment in my physical improvement. There are many. Either some symptom reappears after I thought I was over it or I'm aware of another physical limitation, such as the inability to repair items needing delicate hand control.

I've learned to live with a great many limitations, and things are not as depressing now. One can learn to tolerate a lot of disappointment. As a psychiatrist, I know that one of the best cures for depression is time. Depressions tend to wear off, and there are other things I can do, activities that are more cheerful—a good book, television viewing, and friends. And good things do happen.

At one point I experienced extreme elation. That was the time, about six weeks after the stroke, when someone first recognized my voice on the telephone. It happened twice that day so I knew it wasn't an accident. I was overjoyed and ecstatic—laughing, making jokes, talking. I couldn't be shut up. Several hours later, when I tipped a cab driver $2.50 on a $2.50 fare, I realized I was overreacting. Three days after that I was again delighted when I tried to call home and was able to dial the right number although I didn't have my phone number in my pocket as usual. This time I felt simple pleasure and didn't do anything crazy.

When Zeugma and I discussed my overreaction, he suggested that it might be like an amphetamine "high" and I agreed. Although I've never used amphetamines to the point of getting "high," I have seen many patients who have. It was wonderful, but life isn't all up, and, fortunately, it isn't all down.

The process of recovery is at times one step forward and

two steps back. I've described several regressions, and my dependency was probably the most trying thing for Jane.

Jane: In the early weeks of Clay's illness, I was naturally shocked and frightened, but had little time to think about myself. Clay needed nursing and nurturing and I was eager to do whatever I could. As time went on and he was gradually improving, I occasionally was concerned about his dependency on me, which seemed to be unnecessary. I had no problem about any physical limitations he had, but I wasn't prepared for, nor desirous of, the psychological dependenices. We had always shared chores and responsibilities; each leading a busy life and each respecting and trusting the other. With prolonged illness, this relationship had changed. I made up my mind that I wouldn't allow him to regress, to lose his independence and responsibility.

My choice of a husband had been an independent, strong, at times tyrannical, but definitely capable, head-of-the-household-type. When he was clearly recovering, and Leland's optimism was convincing, I suddenly realized that Clay was dependent on me for the very things I had previously counted on from him—prime financial support, care in case of illness; the kind of person I could look to for taking care of whatever important situations came along.

Apart from my needs, I basically knew that Clay would not benefit from prolonged overindulgence and childlike dependency. It can easily become a habit after the original need no longer exists. Gradually, I started asking him to do certain things, leaving things undone which were previously his domain, acting indecisively, and leaving decisions up to him. At first, he was surprised and then did what was needed. Afterwards we discussed what he could and could not do, and I was delighted each time he added another item to the list of things which were his responsibility. I think he was delighted too. He gradually took over more and more, giving up his passive, regressive "stroke personality."

3

What Happened in Clay's Brain?

A dreadful incident? Yes. Mysterious and incomprehensible? No. Let us try to understand what happened from the neurologist's point of view.

How did Clay know he'd had a stroke? His specialized knowledge played a part, but some of that knowledge is not terribly esoteric. A doctor can examine a patient and pinpoint the site of a stroke because the brain has been mapped out over the course of centuries. The layout is similar for the whole human race, but only similar. The body is like an old house: you know generally the location of the plumbing and electrical lines behind the walls, but they're always in a slightly different place and in a different condition than expected.

The most common cause of stroke is a block in an artery, cutting off blood supply to part of the brain tissue. Deprived of vital oxygen and nourishment, that part of the brain dies. The immediate result depends upon the location of the block. A few elementary facts about the nervous system will make this clear.

Viewed from above, the exposed brain looks like a shelled walnut, divided into two, mirror-image halves. This should not be surprising when we realize that the two halves of our external bodies are also mirror images of each other and that the brain controls the actions of the body. In fact, the surface of the brain contains an actual "map" of the external surface of the body, and we have traced the brain regions which control the mouth, the hand, the leg, the trunk, etc. The brain is also the seat of the mind but is obviously cut off from the external world by the bony skull which encases it. How then can our intellects help us to cope intelligently with the world around us? The brain makes contact with the external world indirectly, via the body.

It is of some interest to consider why both our bodies and brains are constructed as matched mirror-image reflections. Biologists call this layout *bilateral symmetry*. The basic plan is one of the first things a young child learns about anatomy (two hands, two feet, two eyes, etc.). Bilateral symmetry, which we share with most other animals (insects, reptiles, birds, fish, and other mammals), seems to be nature's solution to the problem of efficient design. The problem is an organism's need to move about on the surface of the earth, investigating the environment, seeking food and other pleasures, and avoiding danger. All such creatures are, of course, subjected to the earth's gravity. Forced to acknowledge the distinction between up and down, they develop a top and a bottom which are different; in other words, backs and bellies. At this stage in animal evolution, the mobile creature might be a lowly starfish, possessing a top and a bottom but no special front or rear end, and no right or left sides—just the way a saucer-shaped boat would have no bow, stern, port, or starboard. However, it is more efficient to concentrate most of the intelligent apparatus of the nervous system in a central information center. This would facilitate the making of important decisions in the animal's life especially if the most vital messages about the environment could be routed swiftly and directly to the center, instead of reaching it via some circuitous route. Since one of the most pressing and constant decisions the animal must make is whether or not something is edible, it might be useful to place the information center near the mouth, and to place this part of the body (the head) in front of the other parts. Such strategy would give the creature a competitive edge when there was not enough food to go around, ensuring its survival when its less efficiently designed brethren were starving to death.

Having established a head and tail in addition to a back and belly, nature seems to have shown no great preference for distinguishing the right and left sides of the animal. As it pushes its snout in a continuous search for food, the goodies are just as likely to appear on either side of the body. An efficient solution therefore, is to equip both sides of the body identically so that the creature would be equally prepared for a right or left turn. Thus, we have the basic plan of bilateral, or mirror-image symmetry throughout much of the animal kingdom. It is easier to visualize our proper place in this development when crawling on all fours rather than when walking erect. This down-to-earth position places the human face at the front end of the body and not at the top. Sense organs located at this end of the body have "private lines" to our information center—direct lines to the brain.

If we are to exist effectively in the world, meeting our needs, avoiding danger, and enjoying life, we need information about our environment. This information reaches us through our senses. Vision, hearing, and smell are rather special in this regard. They relay information about objects we are not in immediate physical contact with. The exact location of a distant object is given precisely by eyesight, less precisely by hearing, and only poorly by smell, but all three feed messages directly into the brain. The sense of taste does require a substance to make physical contact with the tongue, but it also has a direct route to the brain.

In contrast, consider our sense of touch which transmits contact information from any part of the body surface. The incoming information is gathered by nerves, microscopic at first, but coalescing progressively into larger and larger cables in the way that tiny rivulets join to form streams, and streams to form rivers. Facial skin, like the senses of sight, sound, smell, and taste, has its private direct route to the brain—the "front end" of a crawling animal is special. For the rest of the body, the coalesced nerve cables converge on the spinal cord at the midline. Unlike the formation of a river, in which the special quality of each contributing stream is obscured by mixing of the waters, the larger cables of the nervous system must preserve information about the source of the messages they are gathering. For example, we want to withdraw the foot which stepped on the tack, not the other one. Or, if the thing we step on happens to feel good rather than painful, we may not want to withdraw the foot at all. As in the case of vision, the location and quality of skin contact remains sorted out in the nervous system in the same way that individual telephone calls gathered in a long-distance cable maintain their identities. The largest cable below the neck is the spinal cord; it finally connects to the brain map in the area where the information reaches our consciousness.

Let's reverse the process. Imagine a message has reached the brain that the right foot itches. The message to scratch it begins in the brain, runs down the spinal cord and out to the hand and arm muscles which will perform the scratching. These outgoing messages follow an opposite but parallel course to the incoming messages—large nerve trunks to progressively smaller ones until they finally narrow down to single microscopic nerve fibers which stimulate individual muscle cells. The final stimulation contracts the muscle which begins the scratching operation. Like incoming messages these outgoing messages from the brain must remain unscrambled. Thus, if we are blindfolded and simultaneously plunge one hand into a bucket of lukewarm water and the other into a bucket of boiling water, only the latter will be withdrawn. The source and destination of incoming and outgoing messages respectively must remain unscrambled in the larger nerve cables (such as the spinal cord) in order that our behavior remain relevant to the real world. The "map" of nerve connections in the brain relates the incoming messsge to the appropriate muscles.

Certain complete reactions can be carried out without ever reaching the brain. If a neurologist taps your knee with a rubber hammer, the knee will jerk via a short-circuit connection located in the spinal cord in the small of the back; the signal need not reach the brain. Under these circumstances the feeling of the hammer tap and the knee jerk would not be conscious. Hence, the derivation of the common metaphor which we use to describe a completely automatic response to a situation—a "knee-jerk reaction."

We have therefore a symmetrical body and a matched symmetrical brain. Each half of the brain contains a map of one-half of the body, and functions as a control center which relates that half of the body to its external environment. As a result of a crisscross of nerves at the base of the brain, each half controls the muscles of, and receives sensation from, the *opposite* half of the body. Although we are not aware of this arrangement consciously, it is very important to the neurologist. He knows that when we are touched on the left half of the body the nerve impulses run up the spinal cord and cross to the right half of the brain. Similarly, a sensation on the right half of the body is registered in the left half of the brain. To move a muscle on the left side of the body a nerve impulse originates in the right half of the brain, crosses over to the left, and runs down the spinal cord to stimulate the appropriate muscle. Similarly, movements of the right side of the body originate in the left half of the brain.

This sequence of nerve impulses is electrochemical, and the critical nerve tissues which conduct the impulses must be maintained constantly by a nourishing blood supply. The supply to the brain is also symmetrical. Each half is nourished by a treelike system of arteries originating in the heart. You can feel the main trunks of these trees pulsing deep in the neck on both sides of your voice box (Adam's apple). As the trunks enter the base of the bony skull they branch repeatedly to reach every part of the brain.

The immediate cause of a stroke usually is a clot (thrombus) which blocks the blood flow in an artery within the brain (cerebrum). Thus, the disease is known as *cerebral thrombosis.* This is to be distinguished from *coronary thrombosis* which is the same sort of thing occurring in an artery supplying the heart muscle—a coronary artery rather than a cerebral artery. These two diseases are closely related in spite of their very different symptoms. When we say that strokes are "usually" due to cerebral thrombosis, we mean eighty percent of all strokes. Another ten percent are due to *cerebral hemorrhage*, a burst or ruptured artery with resultant bleeding into the brain tissue. The remaining ten percent are due to assorted, more esoteric causes.

The riddle of stroke, like the riddle of heart disease, lies in the unsolved problem of aging. Both are due to a deterioration of the body's arterial system—a process known as arteriosclerosis. Sclerosis of an artery can be compared to the aging of a rubber hose. What was originally smooth, elastic, and responsive becomes hard, brittle, and cracked. The edges of the cracks project into the passing bloodstream, and blood clots on the projections. Pieces of these clots tend to break off and become wedged in the progressively narrower channels downstream. Once an artery is blocked, the flow of blood behind the obstruction is stopped, and blood that stands still also clots. Thus, like an auto accident on a narrow road, a small obstruction can cause a huge traffic jam. Brittle hoses also spring leaks, especially when the fluid they conduct is under increased pressure. When a brittle artery in the brain blows out it causes a hemorrhage rather than a thrombosis.

The body's aging does not exactly correspond to the aging of the arterial system. It is true that strokes and heart attacks are quite rare in youth and increasingly common after middle age. Although chronological time passes uniformly for all of us, the age of our plumbing system may differ widely among individuals. Premature sclerosis of the blood vessels tends to run in families. There are also octogenarians with youthful arteries. To complicate matters, the arteries in various parts of the body may not age in uniform fashion. Sclerotic arteries in the limbs occasionally coexist with youthful arteries in the heart and brain, and vice versa.

Amidst all this complexity and ignorance, certain themes or correlations can be discerned. We are sure that diabetes and high blood pressure (the type called "essential hypertension") predispose one to both stroke and heart disease. Diseased hearts are also a notorious source of clots which can break loose only to lodge in an artery of the brain.

Despite the strong connection between arterial deterioration and age, many other aggravating factors in the causation of strokes have been identified, and we can control some of these things. The tendency of blood to clot, so-called "sticky blood," is still highly controversial as a precipitating factor in stroke. Obesity has been implicated in increasing the risk of coronary heart disease, but is apparently unrelated to the incidence of strokes.

"Plaques" are arteriosclerotic areas inside the blood vessels which are literally impregnated with fatty substances, notably cholesterol. A diet low in animal fats is known to lower blood cholesterol, but recent research has shown this factor to be significant only in people under fifty years of age as far as stroke (not heart disease) is concerned. Clay was fifty-five when he was stricken and not overweight, so we cannot honestly say that his adherence to a low cholesterol diet would have made any difference. Smoking is probably related to stroke, as it is to coronary heart disease. Clay was and still is a cigarette smoker.

Only one event has been unequivocally proven to predict a full-blown stroke and that is a *transient stroke*. Clay did not have one. A transient stroke is an attack of diminished blood supply to the brain which results in a localized neurological defect that persists for ten to thirty minutes. The defect may be any localized symptom of stroke, but it must persist for at least this amount of time and then disappear completely within twenty-four hours. Such an attack, especially in males, raises the odds of a severe stroke within a year to 16.5 to 1. Obviously, it is an important warning which requires immediate preventive measures. Episodes of faintness, dizziness, wooziness, transient loss of memory, or inexplicable loss of consciousness do not qualify as transient strokes. Clay's diffuse weakness of the legs on arising in the morning also fails to qualify, although it would have, had the weakness been localized to one leg, persisted for ten to thirty minutes, and then disappeared within twenty-four hours.

Since the brain is encased in a bony skull, doctors have

worked out many ingenious methods of obtaining information short of directly opening the head to take a look. That drastic step is reserved as a last resort. One of the neatest indirect approaches is an examination of the fluid which bathes the brain and the spinal cord—"cerebro-spinal fluid" or CSF. It is a water-clear fluid which is continuously produced in a hollow cavity inside the brain. It normally flows out of this cavity to bathe the surface of the brain, and it leaks down the cavity inside the bony spinal column to bathe the spinal cord. The uninterrupted flow of the fluid surrounding the brain and spinal cord is most fortunate. It is remarkably easy to "tap" the fluid at the base of the spine, but much more difficult to gain access to the fluid inside the skull. Luckily, the spinal fluid is quite representative of the cerebral fluid, thus giving a fair picture of what may be going on in the brain.

The technique is simple and relatively painless. Under local anesthesia a fine, hollow needle is slipped between two of the vertebral bones in the small of the back, until the spinal canal is entered. This entry is signaled by fluid dripping from the outside end of the needle. At this point, a gauge is attached to the needle to measure the pressure of the fluid. The CSF is contained in a bony reservoir, continuously produced and absorbed. Any change in the delicate balance between production and absorption, increasing the former relative to the latter, raises the pressure. In a confined, rigid space the only thing that can give is the brain, so it is important to know about increased pressure as soon as possible in order to avoid brain damage. There are many causes of increased pressure in the CSF. Obviously, any increase in brain volume due to swelling or an expanding tumor, may raise the pressure in the confined reservoir.

In cases of common stroke, however, the spinal tap helps to make an important distinction between a *blocked* artery (thrombosis) and a *burst* artery (hemorrhage) within the brain. The latter is much less common (the ratio is about eight to one) but much more dangerous. A burst artery bleeds into the brain tissue, and eventually the blood reaches the surface of the tissue and leaks into the CSF. The active bleeding not only swells the brain and raises the fluid pressure, but also makes it literally bloody. This is obvious the moment the first drop of fluid comes out of the "spinal tap" needle. The fluid is bloody rather than crystal clear, and if the bleeding is active the pressure is raised. By contrast, an artery which is plugged by a clot—the much more common thrombosis—doesn't bleed. The brain tissue which is deprived of blood may swell somewhat, but the pressure is usually normal and the spinal fluid remains clear. Steroid hormones are now available to reduce the swelling that does occur.

The importance of distinguishing between a thrombosis and a hemorrhage is more than an assessment of the danger of the situation. It bears importantly on possible treatment to be prescribed. In the case of thrombosis, further blockage of the blood supply can be halted by administering drugs which artificially reduce the clotting tendency of the patient's blood. However, if active hemorrhage is in progress, we would not want to interfere with nature's mechanism for stopping the bleeding. Most readers are familiar with the danger of even minor hemorrhage to persons suffering from hemophilia, a genetic defect in the blood clotting mechanism. Since treatment of thrombosis by inhibiting the blood's tendency to coagulate involves making the patient mildly "hemophilic," it is easy to understand why it is critical that the doctor be sure the stroke is not due to cerebral hemorrhage. Clay's spinal tap showed clear fluid under normal pressure and this tended to confirm the diagnosis of thrombosis.

Armed with these facts, we can see how the examining doctor arrives at a probable diagnosis. After getting the complete history of the illness the normal wiring of the nervous system is his key. Imagine that he is confronted with a patient who has muscle weakness on the left side of the body, as well as loss of sensation on the left side. Knowledge of the crisscross arrangement tells the doctor that the stroke has occurred in the right half of the brain. One of the curious antics that comprise the ordinary neurological examination is usually a source of awe and/or amusement, depending upon how sick the patient is. By tickling the sole of each foot and observing the promptness and type of withdrawal response, the neurologist can rapidly test the integrity of both halves of the nervous system. What is he looking for? The normal response is fairly symmetrical. Any asymmetry is cause for suspicion of possible disease.

But one more important fact must be known before we can explain the "Babinski of the left foot" to which Clay made reference. It is the effect of the maturity of the nervous system on the withdrawal response when the sole of the foot is stimulated. A newborn infant finds this type of stimulation just as unpleasant as adults do. There is one important difference, however. When the sole of an infant's foot is tickled, the toes curl *up* as the foot is withdrawn; when the same test is applied to a normal adult, the toes curl *down* during the withdrawal. The infantile pattern develops into the adult pattern as the nervous system matures, roughly when the child begins to walk. This change is believed to stem from the inhibition of the original infantile reaction by the later maturing parts of the brain. It is these same parts of the brain that are damaged by strokes. The result is that the maturation of the nervous system is reversed, so to speak. The adult inhibition of infantile reflexes is removed, permitting them to reappear, or as we say, permitting their release. Yet interestingly, this reversion to the infantile pattern of foot withdrawal—toes curling up instead of down—is only on the side of the body affected by the stroke. This test thus produces a notably asymmetrical response.

When the face, hand, or leg on the same side as the Babinski reflex display weakness and sensation difficulties the opposite half of the brain is implicated. Thus, the classical picture of a stroke such as Clay's includes a Babinski sign on the *right foot.* Here we have a mystery. His Babinski sign was on the left, the wrong side in terms of all the evidence of a left brain stroke. At first we simply discounted Clay's memory of the left-sided Babinski on the first day in the hospital. (After all, he was admittedly confusing the concept of right versus left sides of the body, or the aphasia might have produced the wrong word. However, the neurologist had noted the left Babinski in his hospital chart with enough surprise to attempt an explanation, which he wrote up immediately after the examination. Although complicated, the gist of the explanation is that a shower of tiny, loose plaques from a neck artery on the left can cause massive trouble in the left side of the brain. However, it is conceivable that some people have an unusual connection, and an artery in the left half of the brain may supply some tissue on the right. In such cases, one of the small clots might have crossed to land in the right side of the brain, causing only minor symptoms but producing the surprising left Babinski reflex. In any event, the abnormal reflex was gone on subsequent examinations; the toes of both feet turned down again.

Symptoms of weakness, paralysis, or loss of sensation can be understood by most people from their personal experience. Anyone who has had an injection of novocaine in a dentist's office or whose foot has "fallen asleep" has experienced the type of sensation loss that comes with a stroke. The inability to use muscles is also familiar, at least by analogy to broken arms and legs or sprained ankles. Thus, the symptoms discussed so far can be understood and coped with in terms of common, everyday experience.

Here the plot thickens however. Indeed, if the location of the blocked artery is a matter of chance, what difference if the stroke be right or left? Most people, being right-handed, would probably prefer a left-sided paralysis if forced to choose. There would at least be less interference with normal dexterity, and fewer skills would have to be relearned with the other hand. If this were the only issue, this book would be unnecessary. We now come to the focus of the book, namely, the stroke which interferes with language and speech.

It is perfectly amazing that one of the best documented facts about the brain was not noticed until the early nineteenth century. Brilliant observers have described strokes since antiquity, including the crisscross arrangement, yet had overlooked the obvious fact that right-sided paralysis is often associated with disturbance of speech, whereas left-sided paralysis rarely is. This means that only the left half of the brain controls speech. In this most unique human function the brain is not symmetrical. Therefore, a grim game of Russian roulette is in progress when Fate chooses to afflict one side of the brain. If the blocked artery is in the *left* side, a speech disorder—aphasia—may be added to the symptoms already described.

The symptoms of aphasia are mainly linguistic. There is difficulty in speaking and comprehending speech although general intelligence remains about the same. For literate patients there is also difficulty in reading and writing. But aphasia is mysterious. The difficulty in understanding speech is not due to deafness; hearing is usually normal. The reading problem is not due to blindness; vision is usually unimpaired. The disability specifically involves the deciphering of language. For this reason neurologists have invented terms such as "word deafness" and "word blindness" to distinguish these symptoms from our common understanding of loss of hearing and vision. The same is true for the difficulties in speaking and writing. There may be a mild weakness of the right hand, but not severe enough to account for the disorganization of handwriting. There may be mild weakness of the tongue and muscles around the mouth, but again not severe enough to account for the problem of getting the words out, or for the disorganization of words and sentences that are finally produced.

In the most severe forms of aphasia the patient may be speechless and uncomprehending. More often, some combination of milder symptoms occurs. For example, some speechless patients may comprehend quite well, and demonstrate their understanding by eloquent charades. Others may talk a blue streak but their speech is gibberish; these fluent patients do *not* comprehend the speech of others nor do they seem aware that they aren't getting through. Between these extremes are a bewildering variety of combinations of milder symptoms, several of which characterize Clay's illness.

The outward symptoms of aphasia, no matter how distressing, are merely reflections of some deeper disorder which must be grasped if the reader is to understand Clay's story. How are we to understand this? Is the mind affected? Is the patient mentally defective or unbalanced? No, for communication which bypasses speech, such as pantomime, may reveal normal comprehension. The patient goes about the business of living rationally. He easily carries out many complex nonverbal tasks requiring high intelligence.

It is difficult at first for the average adult to get the feel of an aphasic experience. In principle, we can't know what it's like if we haven't been there ourselves; Clay has been there and returned. There are analogies in everyday life which can provide vicarious participation in Clay's experience. Try the following experiments:

1. Imagine reading these printed words without being able to understand them. No problem with vision, but the words don't seem to mean anything. Haven't we all had this experience while reading ourselves to sleep or with an unfamiliar foreign language that uses the English alphabet? It would be shocking indeed to have this suddenly happen to this very sentence. Yet if it did, we could still copy the words, as any illiterate can, without comprehension. Few of us can remember our preliterate, let alone prespeech, days.

2. Look around and name some object you see, then repeat that name aloud once per second several hundred times while staring at the object. The word becomes a stream of sheer sound which the brain registers but which we tend to ignore when we focus on the meaning.

3. Write the names of all the presidents of the United States, or the names of the fifty states. We assume you'll miss a few. Would you recognize the omissions if you saw them? Of course. Imagine that the names of all the objects in the world were like your omitted items; you couldn't think of the name but could recognize it instantly when someone else said it.

4. Have you ever had a word on the "tip of your tongue"? There are ways to produce the phenomenon. For example, try to remember all the names of people you met at a party or on vacation. When you feel some name is on the "tip of your tongue," try to write down the first letter, the number

of syllables, the rhythm of the name, or something the name rhymes with. When you finally recall the name itself (perhaps with the aid of somebody else), compare it to the guesses you wrote down while it was still on the "tip of your tongue." See how much you knew about a name you couldn't remember! Now imagine speaking this preliminary information without being able to arrive at the final name of anything.

5. Remember a dream in which you heard or spoke a word you understood but had never encountered before. Make up a new word, one that you have never thought about. Where did it come from? Is it similar to some other English words? Why?

6. Now a hard one. Tell a story aloud, something interesting that happened to you recently but which you've never described to anyone. Before you start, turn on your favorite radio news broadcast. Tell the story aloud while listening to the broadcast. Don't be embarrassed. If you have a tape recorder, record the whole thing! Play with the phenomenon of trying to say something interesting and original while listening to the news. Can you speak fluently? Can you comprehend the broadcast? Most people experience a conflict. If they understand the broadcast they find their speech faltering and they may lose the thread of what they're trying to say. Conversely, if they speak fluently and logically the broadcast is reduced to a meaningless stream of sound; it's speech all right but it makes no sense. This conflict between speaking and listening modes, both of which utilize identical systems in the brain, is very close to the aphasic experience.

7. If the former experiment hasn't turned you off, try speaking concurrently with your partner in your next real conversation (pick an understanding, imaginative friend). Why don't people who have something to say to each other say it at the same time? Why do they alternate between speaking and listening? Why does only one person at a time usually have the floor?

8. Recall a time when you approached a door which was clearly marked "Pull" (or "Push") and you automatically did the opposite of the instruction. Transparent glass doors are often marked this way, and it may be the possibility of seeing through the door to the scene beyond that reduces attention

to the instructions. In any event, one often feels foolish carrying out a motion which is the opposite of the one indicated.

These experiments give the reader a few experiences which to the best of our knowledge, are somewhat akin to aphasia. In all these cases the limits of the brain's ability to handle language have somehow been exceeded. Either the mechanism which converts printed text or incoming speech into meaning has gone awry, or the mechanism which converts intended meaning into spoken or written sentences has faltered. If this seems bizarre to the reader, imagine how devastating it must be to the patient.

Aphasia is the cruelest symptom of stroke because it interferes with communication precisely at a time when the patient and his loved ones need it most. Human beings can adjust to almost any situation if they can communicate with others about it. Problems such as paralysis or loss of sensation can be worked out like other problems of living. Aphasics however, cannot work out their problems through the usual channel of conversational ability.

Our story will deal mainly with the left side of the brain, the site of Clay's stroke. Although not talkative, the right side of the brain is far from stupid. This has only been discovered in the last few years as scientists began to study the physical basis of nonverbal forms of intelligence. That nonverbal intelligence exists is pretty obvious to the man in the street, but discoveries in academia often lag behind common sense. It is now known that the right side of the brain is just as specialized as the left. Its special talents include three-dimensional analysis of space, perception of musical and other nonverbal sounds, facial recognition, and the experience of emotion. Thus, compared to its left partner, the right side of the brain is sort of an intellectual low-brow, but the kind that makes life worthwhile. This may account for its long scientific neglect.

Recall that Clay's stroke occurred about 10:00 P.M. when he returned from teaching a course. The course was entitled

Psychophysiology, one of those compound names so fashionable these days. We invent such a new name when two previously loosely related areas of human activity need to be drawn together. His course was about the relationship between the mind and bodily functions. It dealt with the mental and emotional factors in asthma, high blood pressure, stomach ulcers, muscular cramps, skin rashes, heart attacks, and resistance to infection. It also dealt with the psychological problems which such illnesses produce. In short, he was teaching that the mind and body of man are inseparably related, that illness is an illness of the whole person.

It is curious that professionals have to be taught about the unity of body and mind. How did the two ideas get separated in the first place? One suspects that it goes back to the distinction between body and soul; the one mortal and transient, the other immortal and permanent. This split has deep roots in our language. Consider the following contrasts:

Spiritual	versus	Material
Mind	versus	Matter
Theoretical	versus	Practical
Intellectual	versus	Mechanical
Divine	versus	Human
Fantasy	versus	Reality
Psychical	versus	Physical
Knowing	versus	Doing

The words in the right column have a substantial down-to-earth quality which tends to prove itself pragmatically in the tests of daily life. Those on the left must be defended, and often demand great faith. They also tend to be more prestigious, though this value judgment can reverse suddenly, making them seem "fuzzy-headed" and relatively useless. The humanist tradition in both psychiatry and theology finds such distinctions too sharply drawn. In seeking to bridge, blur, or heal the split we invent professional courses with titles such as psychophysiology.

These ancient distinctions have been particularly potent in obscuring the fact that both language and mind are functions of the brain. A case in point is the influence of the famous French philosopher and scientist René Descartes (1596–1650). He was devoted to both Catholicism and scientific method, although the latter was opposed by the churchmen of his day. A personal philosophy resolved his dual allegiance. He began to view the physical world (including the brain) as mechanistic and entirely divorced from the mind; the connection between the two was accomplished by the intervention of God. Descartes' goal, which was to prove the complete independence of man's soul from his body, turned out to be extremely fruitful for the scientific study of the brain. For one thing, it helped brain researchers to avoid being burned at the stake. Unfortunately for psychology and linguistics, however, he had to deal with language in this dualistic view of man. He performed his "judgment of Solomon" as follows: language (reason, concepts, ideas, "internal" speech, meaning) was relegated to the soul; mere articulation (speech) which we share with parrots, and emotional expression which we share with most animals, was relegated to the body. Thus, to the extent that Descartes' division of man is accepted, language and mind cannot be considered an activity of the brain.

This is not an academic argument. In order for human heart, kidney, and liver transplants to be successful, the donor must be pronounced legally dead at the earliest possible moment. The criterion for death can no longer be total cessation of breathing and heartbeat. Such interruption of basic circulation rapidly leads to the death of just the organs to be transplanted, thus defeating the purpose of the whole operation. The criterion is therefore *brain death*. This is determined by an absence of electrical activity in the brain (determined by means of the electroencephalogram) for a period of twenty-four hours. We know that with this amount of brain damage the patient is reduced to a vegetative state. There is no hope for recovery of even a rudimentary level of communicative ability that we could call language, personality, intellect, or awareness of the environment. The patient may still be an effective pump for circulating blood, but is pronounced legally dead as a human being. The decision does not by any means resolve the philosophical issues. But it does establish a working definition of humanity in terms of brain function. The function that has been irrevocably lost is the capacity for human relationships.

Once we equate the concepts of language, mind, and human existence with brain function, we realize that any change of brain function entails another realm of human experience. This includes the brain states which we know popularly as dreams, anxiety, joy, hypnosis, intoxication, and meditation. The argument cuts both ways. To interfere with another person's brain function must, by this equation, infringe upon his humanity. These are controversial matters and somewhat irrelevant to this book. However, they help to make the point that the "aphasic" state, which is a profound alteration of brain function, language, and therefore of mental function, is another valid realm of human experience. One would not want such an experience if it could be avoided, but even unwelcome experiences may be interesting in retrospect.

4

A Look
at Linguistics

I glance out the window and see a terrifying scene. I could summon you so that you'd see it too, instead, I share the experience remotely, by painting a picture in sound. I exclaim, nervously, "A big, fierce dog is chasing a frightened, little child!" Hearing this sentence, you should almost be able to see what I see and feel my emotion. How does this event get transferred from my mind to yours? That is the riddle of language.

What is language? Most people find it difficult to define, a surprising fact inasmuch as they have been using it expertly since childhood. But even an expert driver may be ignorant of what goes on under the hood of a car. As long as communication is adequate we take language for granted; its mechanics are usually unconscious. A special kind of curiosity about the mechanism itself is the province of linguists, who have a compulsion to take it apart and study it. A linguist (from the Latin *lingua* meaning tongue, speech, language) was traditionally a person well-versed in languages, especially those currently in use. The scientific study of language has rendered that definition almost obsolete, and today the term is reserved for those making a serious study of language.

Linguistics has been called the most humanistic of the sciences and the most scientific of the humanities. We are indebted to its practitioners for having specified several important factors in the definition we seek.

Language is a *means of communication*. Communication involves at least a pair of communicators who possess the capability, the opportunity, and the motivation to exchange messages. Pondering this fact, an erudite British neurologist, MacDonald Critchley, was inspired to estimate the number of possible languages. His answer: the world's population divided by two. A less romantic estimate would compute the number of possible conversations if everyone in the world had an opportunity to communicate with everyone else, but the point is clear. People do indeed invent private languages for the purpose of self-communion, but as long as they remain completely private we can't say much about them.

It's unlikely that any means of communication would exist unless there were something important to be communicated in the first place. We need language for communication simply because human experience is subjective and therefore not self-evident. If a child has jam all over her face, some of her recent activities are obvious. However, other factors may not be obvious; for example, the jam may not have been her favorite flavor, or it may have taken twenty minutes to get the jar open. When you see somebody's new sunburn after a holiday, the sheer fact of exposure to the outdoors is silently documented—but not the beauty of a sunset which may also have been part of the event. We need language to communicate personal knowledge that is not obvious; bright ideas, memories, forebodings, private experiences, plans, full bladders, etc. If this wealth of private information showed "like egg on our faces," by telepathy for instance, a casual observer would already know it. Additional communication would be redundant, or would serve some other purpose such as ritual use of language, where the messages are completely predictable. In the immortal words of the lovesick, rejected, hillbilly folksinger, "I can see, hear, feel—I don't have to be told." Language therefore involves communication of some

private experience or some *personal idea* that others cannot immediately share. For example, when a mother gives a baby a
glass of milk they can both see it, feel it, taste it, and smell it.
But when she adds the spoken word "milk" to the event, she
is conveying an aspect of her own experience, the name,
which the child had not yet shared. "Personal" or "private"
refers to some aspect of reality which is present only to oneself; for others to share the experience it must be re-created
for them. It must be "re-presented," that is, made present for
them. The word "milk" is the mother's representation of the
event.

No personal experience can ever be replayed exactly; we
can never "step into the same river twice." Yet we strive for
reasonable facsimiles. In our efforts to re-create a private
event we resort to symbols which *stand for* the original; the
event is represented by means of a code which *takes the place of*
the original. Thus, language is also a *code* which enables us to
re-create our personal experience for others who also know
the code, and who have a roughly equivalent knowledge of
the world.

Codes can be plain or fancy; the degree of similarity between the original idea and the coded message can vary enormously. A huge mountain can be simply represented by a dot
on a map, but a detailed contour map gives more information
about somebody's experience of the mountain. Unlike the
dot, the contour map conveys the experience of steep and
shallow slopes to the veteran hiker or skier; a vicarious experience he might well want to have in preparation for the real
thing. Of course, a three-dimensional scale model represents
the mountain even more accurately than a contour map.
Pushing this argument to its absurd conclusion, the most
faithful map of a mountain is the mountain itself. Unfortunately, like the private experience of another person, it cannot
always be had literally, and is at best an unwieldy representation.

Similarly, a dog may communicate its desire for an outing
by racing to the door while barking excitedly. This behavior
is an actual part of the desired experience. The message is a

partial re-enactment of the event. One can teach the dog to pick up its leash before racing to the door, since this "trick" is also an integral part of the experience of the outing, although not a natural part of a dog's behavior.

Animal training is as old as civilization, but it took the Russian psychologist, Ivan Pavlov, to make it a part of twentieth century science. His classic experiment showed that a *completely arbitrary* signal could be made to symbolize a natural stimulus in the animal's world. The sight and smell of food naturally causes a hungry dog to salivate as it prepares to devour and digest the forthcoming meal. A ringing bell produces no such reaction. Pavlov began to ring a bell whenever food was presented to a hungry dog. Eventually, the dog salivated when it heard the bell—even in the absence of food. This experiment was a clear demonstration that the normally unappetizing sound of a bell had come to represent food to the dog's nervous system. The choice of a bell as a code for the food experience is arbitrary; a buzzer or a flash of light would have served just as well. Codes which bear no necessary relation to the events they represent are abstract.

There are many different types of codes. Road signs are analogues for the driving conditions to be anticipated, and are not usually arbitrary symbols. A cross depicts an intersection; a "Y" shape a fork in the road. Curves ahead are signalled by a wavy line, and a representation of children playing means just that.

Now contrast the following illustration. Many youngsters have sent boxtops away to receive a secret coding device from Dick Tracy or Little Orphan Annie. They receive a pair of concentric discs joined through their centers by an axle so that they can be independently rotated. One disc has the alphabet printed around its rim, evenly spaced so that A follows Z. The other disc contains the corresponding numbers 1 through 26. The secret code is produced by a key; for example, the key "A1" means "set the letter A opposite the number 1." Then of course, 2 means B, 3 means C, and so on. Knowing the key to the code permits the child to decipher the numerical message 4, 1, 14, 7, 5, 18 as the word "danger."

In the "A1" code:
4 means D
1 means A
14 means N
7 means G
5 means E
18 means R

If the device were reset to another code whose key is "A3," 3 now means A, 4 means B, etc. When we reach 26 (X) 1 then means Y and 2 means Z. Now the same message ("danger") is conveyed by a different sequence of numbers.

In the "A3" code:
6 means D
3 means A
16 means N
9 means G
7 means E
20 means R

This penny gadget has provided generations of children with a sense of high adventure, and has exasperated their younger siblings who were not let in on "the secret." It has also sold a lot of breakfast cereal. It may also have been an early inspiration for certain professional cryptographers, providing their first insight into the arbitrary nature of many language codes. Edgar Allan Poe used this insight in "The Gold Bug." Note what little difference it makes which code is used (there are 26 possibilities —"A1" to "A26"), it is completely arbitrary. One only needs to know the spelling of the English word, the numbers, and the convention (rule or key) which relates letters to numbers. Using the key to transform a word into numerals is called *encoding;* the reverse process is called *decoding.* As long as the encoder and decoder both speak English and agree about the key, they can communicate their ideas about the world numerically.

We are dwelling on the arbitrary, conventional quality of some language codes for a particular reason. Language loss in aphasia, as well as subsequent recovery, may have much to do with the type of connection between the symbol and the idea to be symbolized; that is, with the nature of the code itself. The language of pantomime, for example, uses gestures which are themselves part of what is being expressed. In contrast, words are much more arbitrary, assigned to the ideas they represent purely by convention and general agreement. The words "dog," "chien," and "hund" all refer to the same animal, yet none is more descriptive of the animal than the other. Speech is an abstract code compared to mime; they are very different types of language.

A passing nod of acknowledgment should be given to theories of phonetic symbolism, which document many cases where the word chosen to represent an experience does indeed bear some relation to the real event. The poetic mechanism of onomatopoeia is one such example. The name "bee" may be arbitrary, but perhaps not the word "buzz." The theory becomes stronger when words are found in historically unrelated languages which express some common idea by means of a particular sound. It is noted, for instance, that words for "mother" in many languages have an "m" sound, presumably related to the instinctual sucking gesture of breast feeding. Words expressing negation in many languages have a nasal sound accompanied by a wrinkling of the nose, similar to the disgust gesture produced by a bad taste or odor. It may be that the characterization of speech as a purely arbitrary system must be qualified somewhat. The fact remains however, that sound symbolism is impossible to demonstrate for at least ninety-nine percent of the words on this page.

Another important feature of language is its grammar. This is one of the most fascinating facts about language: the speaker's intuition (when using their native tongue) is the best test of whether a given statement conforms to or violates the rules of that language. This is true even if the speaker is naive, and cannot verbalize the rules. Let's try a few gross examples:

1) "glimp" is a possible English word; "lgimp" is not.
2) "The green hat" is a possible English phrase; "The hat green" is not.

3) "The man was astonished" sounds right; "The rock was astonished" does not.

4) "Hello" is an appropriate greeting; "Goodbye" is generally not.

Linguists spend their lives working out the precise rules that are used in these examples. Yet an illiterate speaker of English will detect the strangeness of the second half of all four illustrations. The response may be amusement or disbelief but the anomaly is noticed. Intuition is a reliable criterion even when the native user cannot describe exactly what is wrong. Even aphasics who have lost the power of intelligible speech may nevertheless be capable of distinguishing appropriate patterns from nonsensical ones in their native language.

A language mediates between private ideas and the public messages which transmit those ideas. A mediator is a go-between, without special loyalty to either of the parties involved. A mediator's job is to establish a relationship or an agreement that benefits both parties. A grammar, which is the structure of a language code is similar. The purpose of language is to transmit an idea that is private; the transmission requires an overt signal, a public message. The overt signal can be totally arbitrary; beeps, gestures, ink marks on a page, or vocal noises, all essentially devoid of intrinsic meaning. The actual signal may indeed be an interesting pattern, perhaps decorative, but otherwise as unintelligible as Egyptian hieroglyphs were prior to the discovery of the Rosetta stone. The power of an overt message to convey an idea from one mind to another requires that both sender and receiver share a roughly equivalent knowledge of the world, as well as an identical grammar.

The grammar of a language is scientifically described in terms of a *finite number of discrete elements* plus a *finite number of rules* for their combination. "Finite" means that there are limits or boundaries. However, we shall see that grammar is capable of expressing an infinite number of ideas, because new ideas can always be produced. How does such a grammar work?

At the opening of this chapter we examined the sentence

"A big, fierce dog is chasing a frightened, little child!" The speaker's initial view of the scene and instant grasp of its significance was, from the viewpoint of the impending sentence, nonverbal. It presupposed extensive knowledge of the world: what a dog is; that fierce dogs bite; that certain facial expressions express fear and the desire for escape; that big creatures often pursue small ones; etc. Also, in the split second before the sentence formed in the speaker's mind, there was a sense of fear and a need to tell someone about it, perhaps to have the listener do something about it. The roots of speech therefore include extensive nonverbal world knowledge, emotion, intention, and a human relationship that encompasses these experiences.

The sentence indicates that at least six major preverbal ideas struck the speaker, perhaps simultaneously:

1. dog chase child   (The dog chases the child.)
2. dog big   (The dog is big.)
3. dog fierce   (The dog is fierce.)
4. child little   (The child is little.)
5. child frightened   (The child is frightened.)
6 scary scene   (I am scared.)

A photo of the event would implicitly embody all these ideas. They are rendered above in pidgin English to suggest their primitive, preverbal quality; they also suggest the various propositions that get woven into the sentence finally uttered. The first states the main event, the actors, and the relation between them. The next four propositions indicate qualities of the actors and are used as descriptive adjectives in the resultant sentence. The last is a statement about the observer and is conveyed by the nervous tone of voice rather than by words. The phrasing, the intonation, and perhaps the rhythm of the sentence, may be sensed by the the speaker prior to the precise choice of words, as when trying to recall a poem that is "on the tip of the tongue." As the words take form they constitute a set of commands to the speech muscles which produce the sequence of consonants and vowels which we recognize as speech. This progression from meaning to sound is roughly reversed in the listener, whose analytic task is to impose a sensible interpretation upon the sound sequence. In the optimal case the meaning arrived at is identical to that intended. This page is another version of the speech code.

The smallest elements of the speech code are roughly the vowels and consonants—forty-six sounds in all for spoken English. This number is finite partly because of our limited ability to hear differences; some sound variation is too slight to be noticed. The same word is never spoken twice in precisely the same way, and the acoustics of a room can cause huge variations that we routinely disregard. But more interesting is the tendency of our hearing apparatus to make decisions when situations are truly ambiguous. For example, the consonants "p" and "b" are produced in exactly the same way except for a buzzing of the vocal cords in the latter case. With special equipment in the acoustic laboratory, it is now possible to vary the intensity of this distinguishing buzz and produce a continuous gradation of the physical sound pattern between these two consonants. The listener however, doesn't hear anything as ambiguous as an intermediate consonant between "p" and "b." The psychological experience is more of an abrupt jump from one consonant to the other at some intermediate point. This tendency to hear categories further limits the sound variations that matter, restricting them to the finite number of discrete sounds that we actually perceive as different. In the case of vowels, which are more musical than consonants, the situation is a bit more fluid; we can hear continuous variation between vowels (the cat's "meow" is an example) but we still identify only a finite number of vowels.

These basic sound units are then combined, according to a finite number of rules, to form a finite number of syllables. Each syllable usually has its own vowel, and the monosyllabic word "a" is just that. A consonant can be tacked on before a vowel ("to"), after a vowel ("at"), or in both places ("tat"). Consonants can also occur in clusters: the monosyllabic word "splits" has three consonants preceding the vowel and two following it. Certain difficulties in speaking after a stroke occur during attempts to produce complex syllables.

For reasons buried in history, the rules of English permit certain sound sequences, such as words beginning with "pl" (place), but prohibit others, such as words beginning with "lp," or "ng." However, a word can end with "lp" (help) or "ng" (sing). And the word "nga" can be heard in West Africa. Many of the prohibited sound sequences in a given language can actually be articulated in infancy, but seem to undergo atrophy and can no longer be produced accurately by a native speaker. This accounts for persistent foreign accents when one attempts to learn a second language later in life, such as the native English speaker's problem with the French vowel sound "tu," or the "umlaut" sound in German (ö), or the native Chinese speaker's substitution of "l" for "r" in English. Other prohibited sound sequences, though quite easy to pronounce—words beginning with "zl" in English for example—somehow never come to mind. "Zilch" is a possible English word but "zlich" isn't. Thus, when preschool children invent nonsense words, which they do all over the world, the sound sequences conform to the rules of their native language.

Many single syllables are already complete words, and a change of only one of their consonants or vowels completely changes the meaning. Compare the effect of a vowel change in the syllables "pat, pet, pit, pot, put"; or the effect of an initial consonant change in the syllables "bit, pit, lit, sit, kit, tit, wit, fit, hit"; or the effect of a final consonant change in the syllables "bid, big, bin, bit."

Other syllables function as complete units of meaning but cannot stand alone as words; they must be attached to other meaningful syllables. The syllable "un" for example, serves to negate (unbend, undo, unreel), and one of its combination rules is that it must be a prefix. Yet there are words which it cannot negate (nouns), which accounts for the humorous effect of Lewis Carroll's "unbirthday." The syllable "ness" is another example; it converts adjectives to nouns as in kindness, happiness, or ugliness. Its combination rules require that it be a suffix. One knows intuitively that some rule is being violated when "ness" is attached to nouns (chairness, treeness, etc.) even though the meaning of such words may be clear, as in the case of "unbirthday." Still other syllables have no independent meaning (ji, ga, ef) but enter into the composition of larger meaningful units (jinx, gab, effort).

To recapitulate, there is a finite inventory of distinguishable sounds in a language, and a finite number of rules for stringing these sounds together into permissible sequences called syllables. The finite inventory of syllables is larger than that of sounds, and is the basis from which words are constructed. Many words are single syllables. Longer words are governed by a larger, but still finite number of rules for syllable combination. Words comprise the mental dictionary. At any given time the dictionary is also of finite size, although it can be expanded by learning or inventing new words.

As soon as one begins to discuss sound sequences that are meaningful rather than nonsensical, the roles they play in larger statements become important. For example, the word "pet" standing alone is terribly ambiguous. It can be an adjective, a noun, or a verb; one can "pet a pet pet." Only the surrounding context can make sense of the word intended. Thus, we have the next level of language organization—the rules for combining the dictionary elements into phrases.

Isolated phrases make more sense than isolated words, but still constitute primitive utterances; "the pet" can be the subject of the sentence "*The pet* is hungry," or the object of the sentence, "He fed *the pet*." The next level of the language hierarchy consists of the rules for combining phrases into permissible sentences. In the progression from the smallest meaningful sound sequence to words, phrases, and sentences, we begin to recognize syntax, the rules which specify how words can be combined to produce well-formed statements.

A well-formed statement doesn't have to make sense. For example, the following sentence is syntactically correct; it has a subject, verb, and object. "The decomposed antelope unzipped the fierce saucer." What is wrong with this sentence? Utilizing naive intuition, one might imagine a scenario which rationalizes the sentence. Out of context, "the decomposed antelope" makes sense since dead antelopes rot. One can then say, "The decomposed antelope was unpleasant." "The fierce saucer" is more problematical. Inanimate objects generally don't have emotions, but the ceramist who produced this particular saucer may have been a creative type who made the saucer look really fierce. We could then understand the sentence: "The ceramist created the fierce saucer." This proves that "the fierce saucer" can be the appropriate object of a transitive verb. However the verb "unzipped" creates more of a problem. It certainly is a transitive verb, which means it has a subject which does the unzipping and an object which gets unzipped. How can the fierce saucer be unzipped? Any ceramist wild enough to create a fierce saucer might well put a zipper on it; "pop art," so to speak. We can now believe that, "The ceramist unzipped the fierce saucer." We are however, still left with the problem of the decomposed antelope. Whoever or whatever unzips a zipper must be in a condition to accomplish such an action. Even assuming that antelopes can be trained to unzip things, how can a decomposed antelope manage it? This has gone far enough to make the linguist's point: there are sentences which are syntactically perfect and semantically anomalous.

We've just seen that a syntactically correct sentence can be nonsensical unless interpreted metaphorically. If decomposition, for example, didn't imply death, but was a metaphor on the state of health, the sentence would be meaningful by a stretch of the imagination. However, if the same sentence is rendered, "Antelope the decomposed unzipped fierce the saucer," it makes even less sense than before. Scrambling of the word order prohibits even a farfetched metaphorical interpretation.

There is therefore intuitive evidence for some independence between syntax and semantics. What is the origin of such an idea? The distinction between form and content is ancient and obvious. There is the container and that which is contained. A vessel, whether filled with milk, water, wine, or sand, imparts its shape to the contents indiscriminately. A statue can be cast in a variety of metals; a penny can be changed from copper to steel to relieve a shortage of imported materials. Conversely, water remains water whether in a liquid, solid, or gaseous state. Personal identity survives transformation of physical form from birth to old age. Both God and the Devil can appear in different guises. A magician makes things disappear, but they don't cease to exist.

Depending on the example chosen, either form or substance remains immutable while the other varies. Both have independent existence, and the ancient dichotomy exists in linguistics as a split between syntax and semantics. Although the issues are complex and controversial, there does seem to be a division in the mental dictionary between the essential substantive words of a message and those words which comprise the syntactic glue that joins these meaningful items. It is best seen in the composition of telegrams and headlines.

A message needs to be sent, each word is costly and brevity is essential. What part of the message may safely be omitted? Language knowledge dictates a strategic economy; the small grammatical words get dropped. The headline "Boy, Dog, Saved" is produced by deleting five words from the sentence, "The boy and his dog have been saved." These expendable words are called function words because they often lack a clear referential meaning in themselves. They serve to indicate the grammatical relationship between the retained items in the telegrammatic message. They include prepositions, articles, auxiliaries, and perhaps pronouns. These words tend to be unaccented when spoken, or unstressed as linguists say. The abbreviated message consists of content words which have independent referential meaning and include nouns, verbs, and adjectives. These words tend to be accented; they receive greater stress. If provided only with content words we can usually fill in the function words, but obviously we can't do the reverse. A telegram composed of function words would be relatively meaningless.

A surprising fact about conversational speech is not generally appreciated; namely that almost half of all the words spoken are chosen from a list of thirty words, almost all of them function words. In the authors' previous research on three million words in psychotherapy interviews, these words, in descending order of frequency, were:

I, and, to, the, that, of, it, you, was, know, a, me, in, it's, but, well, think, like, have, don't, about, or, just, I'm, when, at, so, what, do, as

With so few items accounting for almost half of all speech the well-known redundancy of our language is not surprising. Deletion of these function words produces the succinct, pithy quality of telegrams and headlines.

The ability of language users both to produce and understand messages in telegrammatic style is a powerful argument for a basic distinction between syntax and semantics. But the origin of this ability, which appears virtually spontaneously without special tutelage, still demands explanation. The explanation may be no farther away than the nearest two-year-old child. The earliest sentences produced during language acquisition are indeed in telegrammatic style. "See car, more milk, Jimmy go bye-bye, baby sleepy, big doggie, nice dollie, Mommy come home," are some examples. Adults all have the ability to "baby-talk" in this fashion. So the source of this ability may be found in original childhood grammar—the manner in which every one of us begins to speak. Telegrammatic speech is also an important feature in certain aphasic disorders.

There are obvious limits to telegrammatic style. Word order is a major clue to syntax since the subject of actions generally precedes the verb whereas objects of actions follow: "Mitzi found Lulu." But our grammar permits a passive construction: "Lulu was found by Mitzi." Part of language knowledge consists of realizing that these two sentences mean the same thing. Yet deletion of function words from the second yields "Lulu found Mitzi," which is the opposite of the intended meaning. This, of course, brings us to the essential function of the grammar; making sense of what we hear and saying what we mean.

At the level of sheer sound sequence, an individual suffering from a head cold may say "beople," and the listener knows that the intent must have been "people" since the word spoken does not exist. A more problematical sentence might be: "He gave me a bat on the head." Here, accurate decoding depends on context outside the sentence since both "bat" and "pat" are possible. Is an affectionate encounter being described? If so, the rules of connected discourse make the interpretation "bat" improbable though not impossible.

The phrases "white shoes" and "why choose" when spoken quickly have virtually identical sound patterns. Yet they could never be confused when used in the following sentences: "He wore white shoes." "I like them both, so why choose?" An intuitive sense of propriety tells us that the following alternative interpretations are probably nonsense. "He wore why choose." "I like them both, so white shoes." The alternatives violate syntactic rules and are consequently untenable. Another sound sequence which is ambiguous when spoken rapidly is described by the following two sentences: "The good can decay many ways." "The good candy came anyways." In this case, both versions are semantically and syntactically acceptable in isolation. Only the larger context of the narrative in which they are used can assign the intended meaning.

In the two preceding examples the very words being spoken were ambiguous until used in a larger context. Equally interesting are isolated sentences in which all the words are absolutely clear, but which necessitate more than one reading: "They are flying planes." This sentence can be an answer to the question, "What are they doing?" In that event, "flying" is a verb. It could also answer the question, "What kind of planes are they?" In that case, "flying" is an adjective. The grammatical structure in the speaker's mind is obviously dependent on which reading is intended; unfortunately, grammar is covert. Both meanings happen to yield the identical overt message, forcing the reader to decide between them on the basis of other criteria. Another example of such ambiguity is: "I like her cooking." This might mean that I like her when she is engaged in the act of cooking; that I like the things that she cooks; or, by some stretch of the imagination, that I like the fact that she is being cooked. Here, three completely different grammatical structures, corresponding to the three readings, could be operating in the mind of the speaker. Yet all of them produce the identical overt message. Again, effective communication of meaning must appeal to the broader context of the discourse.

As a final example, our intuitive understanding of syntax tells us that the following two sentences may mean the same thing: "The policeman found the baby." "The baby was found by the policeman." However, we cannot be sure because the second sentence is ambiguous. The word "by" may have the meaning, "in the vicinity of," as in: "The baby was found by the swimming pool."

We have described a hierarchical organization of the grammatical system, ascending from sounds to syllables, words, phrases, and sentences. At each level in the hierarchy there is a collection of elements and rules for their combination and use.

A critical change occurs above the phrase level. We refer to the emergence of a feature that converts a pedestrian grammar into a "new sentence factory." It makes possible the expression of an infinite number of ideas by means of a finite number of elements and rules. It accounts for the creativity of language in the sense that we can say something which we have never heard before, and comprehend something we have never said or even thought about. Recall that below the level of the sentence, everything in the language can be listed—actually written down—and is therefore finite. It is possible to list the forty-six English sounds and all their permissible syllable combinations. One can also list the whole mental dictionary, which is only a small proportion of the more than half-million entries in *Webster's Unabridged Dictionary*, which in turn is fewer than the finite number of words in the English language. It is also feasible to write down all the possible phrases that could be constructed from these basic materials, although it might certainly consume the lives of an army of linguists, even with the aid of high speed computers. It is however, impossible to list all the conceivable sentences in a language for a reason that might at first, seem trivial. The argument takes the form of an easily understandable mathematical proof; namely, the proof that there are an infinite number of whole numbers. The proof goes as follows: pick any whole number (an integer), for instance 7 or 999 or 100,662. Regardless of the number selected, the rules of arithmetic permit the addition of the number 1. Thus, for any number selected, there is always a larger one—meaning there is no end to the process.

Using the same type of reasoning one can prove that there is an infinite number of sentences in the language. For example,

This is the house that Jack built.
This is the malt that lay in the house that Jack built.
This is the rat that ate the malt that lay in the house that Jack built.
This is the cat that ate the rat that ate the malt that lay in the house that Jack built.

The process could go on indefinitely because a phrase can be used again and again. Thus, for any given sentence, a longer one can be constructed which includes the original. Since the longer one is always a slightly different sentence, there is no limit to the number of original sentences that can be constructed.

There's no denying the truly mystical experience that attends the recognition of an endless horizon. Most children realize at some point that they can go on counting indefinitely, and the emotion is one of awe. The human soul is never freer than when contemplating the infinite. Thus, it is tempting to discover the creative possibilities of a language whose finite dictionary and finite number of rules can produce an infinite number of sentences.

For example, the final sentence of the previous paragraph may never have been said before in exactly those words. This certainly defines some low level of creativity despite the fact that the sentence in question is a mere paraphrase of a current idea. The fact that a novel sentence can always be manufactured seems very basic insurance against the risk that civilization will get caught in an intellectual rut. But beyond that, one would hope that the creative possibilities of language produce novel sentences or ideas by virtue of beauty, truth, or wisdom—and not simply length. A trite expression in a novel context can, at times, be more creative than a genuinely new, though trivial, remark. The word "creative," with its connotation of esthetic value over and above mere novelty, may be too loaded a word to apply to this emergent aspect of grammar; perhaps "productive" is a more appropriate term.

The speaker's ability to produce genuinely novel sentences using a standard kit of grammatical tools finds its counterpart in the listener's ability to comprehend them. It is indeed wondrous that any speaker can utter an original statement never before heard in the history of the human race. It is equally wondrous that another person instantly understands what the statement means. The explanation lies in the fact that conversational partners share a common grammar; the identical kit of tools is employed in producing and understanding utterances—in encoding and decoding.

The need to account for the production and comprehension of novel utterances has radically altered our conception of the nature of language knowledge in the past two decades. If the originality and potentially unlimited variety of utterances is taken into account, surely learning a language cannot entail the literal learning of its sentences. Rather, the acquisition of a language must entail learning the elements—sounds, syllables, words—and their rules of combination. All valid statements in the language—past, present, and future—could then be handled. A child unconsciously acquires an implicit knowledge of grammar—a general purpose mechanism. Acquiring a language involves the development of an implicit theory of that language.

This becomes less mysterious when compared to the learning of tennis. The elements include a serve, forehand, backhand, etc., and they are combined according to the rules of the game. Since any rally can go on indefinitely, as can any deuce game or deuce set, virtually every game is unique. In much the same way, a sentence never before spoken can always occur. Learning the game of tennis involves learning the basic strokes and rules which can generate any game that might transpire. Someone with knowledge of the game (the language) can tell when a valid match is being played even though that particular match may not exactly correspond to any other previously witnessed.

Of course, knowing the game, even being able to referee a match, is not the same as being able to play a match. In tennis there is another level of knowledge of the game which also illustrates the general principles of language knowledge. Developing a backhand does not entail learning a fixed stroke, but rather the sequence of movements which, in combination, will lead to a fair return of the ball from the backhand position. The ball never approaches twice in exactly the same way, nor is the player ever in precisely the same position. Although all backhand shots have much in common, each represents some unique configuration of ball, court, player, opponent, game, set, and match, which influences its precise manner of execution. We can play (or appreciate) tennis to the extent that we understand all the elements that each stroke depends on. There are too many influences to be learned in detail; we must be able to make decisions on the basis of general principles which constitute the implicit knowledge of this acquired skill.

We complete the hierarchy of language where we began it—in the service of its ultimate goal, human communication. The rules of connected discourse and conversation have not yet been formalized by linguists. The rules of discourse might include the notion of a general topic or point to be made, although people do occasionally chatter for no other apparent purpose than to hear the sounds of each others' voices. A conversation in which every sentence involved a change of topic would certainly be violating some rule of discourse. Conversation, of course, decrees that speaker and listener must alternate; only one person has the floor at a time. Concurrent speech and comprehension is virtually impossible, although some specially gifted simultaneous translators seem to have acquired the knack.

It is unfortunate that the most critical level of the hierarchy is the one we know least about. Most attempts to delimit language knowledge have tended to end the analysis of the linguistic system at the level of the sentence. Yet, there is growing evidence that a correct understanding of sentence production cannot divorce itself from the role of the sentence in connected discourse, or the role of connected discourse in actual conversation, or the role of conversation in human relationships. On repeated occasions in this chapter, some difficulty of interpretation at one level of the linguistic system ceased to be a problem when the enveloping context was considered. This suggests, for example, that just as sound ambiguity can be resolved by considering words, word ambiguity by considering sentences, and sentence ambiguity by considering connected discourse, discourse ambiguity may be resolved by considering conversations, and in particular, the communicative relationship between the participants. This raises the possibility that a future theory of language may have to involve the users' general knowledge of the world, and cannot be restricted to a study of linguistic facts as presently conceived. The implication is that distinctions between syntax and semantics, and between language knowledge and its practical use for communication, will some day be considered somewhat artificial. A few illustrations may make this clear.

The sentence "I like her cooking," when isolated, is subject to all the amusing ambiguity described previously. However, "This tastes delicious, I like her cooking," or "She's keeping busy, I like her cooking," or "Leave her in the pot, I like her cooking," goes far in resolving the ambiguity in the isolated sentence. Furthermore, these prefatory sentences may themselves be redundant if the listener can glean the context from nonverbal information. Is the speaker watching somebody in the kitchen, tasting the food after it is cooked, stirring a pot with a dead woman in it, or (metaphorically) commenting upon the fact of a female being maintained in some agonizing emotional state? The alternative interpretations of an isolated ambiguous sentence usually catalogue the variety of conversational contexts in which it could appropriately fit.

Another kind of context is the relative emphasis given to different syllables in a spoken utterance, not usually indicated in print. "He greeted her and then she insulted him." This appears to be a syntactically well-formed sentence, and it makes sense semantically when emphasized "He greeted her and then she INSULTED him." However, the same sentence can be spoken: "He greeted her and then SHE insulted HIM." In this case, the sentence is well-formed only if greeting is an insult; otherwise, the stress pattern makes no syntactic sense. Such sentences seem to say that syntax and semantics are not quite as independent as other examples might lead one to believe.

It is also not yet clear where the division between linguistic and nonlinguistic knowledge is to be drawn, if it can be drawn at all. In a conversation between a trout fisherman and a banker it may be evident that when discussing a bank they are referring to a place where money is deposited and not the side of a stream. Yet, it is likely that the connotation of the word is quite different for each of them. Finally, there is considerable evidence that study of the conversational contexts in which language is actually used can both resolve apparent problems in the theory of language and create new ones. This conversational matrix is of ultimate importance to us inasmuch as aphasia is, in the final analysis, a disease of verbal intercourse. In following chapters we will see what light the language disorders which result from brain disease can throw on these linguistic questions.

5

Language and the Brain

Neurolinguistics is a newcomer to medical research. Traditional linguists worked with perfected, textbook versions of languages such as French, or now-dead languages like Sanskrit. That the language was manufactured by living brains and performed a practical function in the lives of its users was considered peripheral or irrelevant. But language is rarely found in its perfect form and communication failures occur with alarming frequency. At such times we need to know the underlying neural mechanisms to fully understand what went wrong.

Patients are usually content to accept doctors' technical explanations uncritically. In the jungle we must trust the guide. But how do we know that language depends heavily upon the left half of the brain, indeed, upon the brain at all? It may be of interest to see how the neurologist can explain a fact which bears no relation to subjective experience.

Prior to the nineteenth century, linguistics was less a science than a somewhat unsystematic intellectual pursuit by learned individuals who were occasionally also physicians. Such individuals were in a fortuitous position to make impor-

tant, pioneering observations. Another historical reference
source was literary individuals who became stroke victims,
and who commented on the change in their language skills.

On Monday the 16 I sat for my picture, and walked a considerable way with little inconvenience. In the afternoon and evening I
felt myself light and easy, and began to plan schemes of life. Thus I
went to bed, and in a short time waked and sat up as has long been
my custom, when I felt confusion and indistinctness in my head
which lasted, I suppose about half a minute; I was alarmed and
prayed God, that however he might afflict my body he would spare
my understanding. This prayer, that I might try the integrity of my
faculties I made in Latin verse. The lines were not very good, but I
knew them not to be very good, I made them easily, and concluded
myself to be unimpaired in my faculties.

Soon after I perceived that I had suffered a paralytick stroke, and
that my Speech was taken from me. I had no pain, and so little
dejection in this dreadful state that I wondered at my own apathy,
and considered that perhaps death itself when it should come, would
excite less horrour than seems now to attend it.

In order to rouse the vocal organs I took two drams. Wine has
been celebrated for the production of eloquence; I put myself into
violent motion, and, I think, repeated it. But all was vain; I then
went to bed, and, strange as it may seem, I think, slept. When I saw
light, it was time to contrive what I should do. Though God
stopped my speech he left me my hand, I enjoyed a mercy which
was not granted to my Dear Friend Laurence, who now perhaps
overlooks me as I am writing and rejoices that I have what he
wanted. My first note was necessarily to my servant, who came in
talking, and could not immediately comprehend why he should read
what I put into his hands.

I then wrote a card to Mr. Allen, that I might have a discreet
friend at hand to act as occasion should require. In penning this note
I had some difficulty, my hand, I knew not how nor why, made
wrong letters. I then wrote to Dr. Taylor to come to me, and bring
Dr. Heberden, and I sent to Dr. Broclesby, who is my neighbour.
My Physicians are very friendly and very disinterested, and give me
great hopes, but you may imagine my situation. I have so far recovered my vocal powers, as to repeat the Lord's Prayer with no very
imperfect articulation. My memory, I hope, yet remains as it was.

But such an attack produces solicitude for the safety of every Faculty.[2]

The point is that these anecdotal observations were casual. They were not wholesale attempts to systematize the relation of language to brain function. This was partly due to the undeveloped state of both disciplines; the scientific study of both language and the nervous system has really blossomed since the nineteenth century. But another reason for our prolonged ignorance of the physical basis of language is a curious quirk of bodily experience; namely, that of all the organs in the body the brain alone is insensitive. Surgery on the brain itself, once the skull has been opened, does not require anesthesia. The patient is comfortable and fully conscious. It follows that we cannot experience the brain's activity in the place that it occurs—inside the head itself. Rather, the activity of the brain is referred to the source and destination of its messages. This is dramatically demonstrated when a neurosurgeon gently stimulates the exposed brain to map its functions prior to removal of selected diseased tissue. The patient may experience flashes of light, sounds, voices, or complete visual scenes, but these are experienced in the environment rather than in the head. Stimulation of certain locations while the patient is speaking causes acceleration or cessation of speech. The patient is aware of these effects but cannot account for them, being unaware of the stimulus. In short, we don't experience brain events where they occur but rather how they effect our lives and our surroundings. This could account for the long delay in realizing that language is a brain function.

Where is the boundary of the body? Most of us would probably vote for the skin surface, but that isn't the psychological reality. When the dentist anesthetizes one half of our jaw it feels much larger than the unanesthetized side. A blind man's body extends to the end of his cane. When parking an automobile we "feel" for the curb with the car's front tire. A

2. From Samuel Johnson's *Letter 4*. Third day of illness. (850 Chapman collection.) To Mrs. Thrale, in Bath, June 19, 1783.

painter's skill is in the tip of his brush. When we take off a pair of ice skates, there is a soft cushion between the soles of our feet and the ground. These are not metaphors; they are very real physical experiences. Instruments which serve as extensions of the body enlarge the body image, and others recognize this fact. Recall how people tended to give Clay a wide berth when he carried a cane. We locate important events at the interface between our egos and the environment. And our egos are not limited by our skins. This is the work of the brain, itself insensitive, projecting the boundaries of the body image to where the action is.

Can we then understand the old punishment administered to children for speaking profanity—washing their mouths out with soap? Or a music master striking a pupil on the fingers to correct a note played out of tune? Or the expression, "See no evil, hear no evil, speak no evil." Surely, evil must first be seen and heard before it is understood to be evil and it must be understood before it can be unspoken. Yet, folklore locates all these events in the mouth, the fingers, the eyes, and the ears—all essentially supplementary servants of the brain.

Where is speaking skill located? Common sense places it in the mouth. When groping for a word which we can't remember, it is often said to be "on the tip of the tongue," because that's just the way it feels. Most people won't believe that the problem is in the brain and not in the mouth because it doesn't feel that way. Let's examine several other examples of the everyday experience of trying to locate a complex skill.

When first learning to play the piano, write, type, or knit, one's whole being seems to be engaged in the task. The neck or back may become stiff with tension, and the tongue may stick out. Total concentration and undivided attention are required during the first painful steps of the learning process. But with continued practice, the task becomes easier and eventually, automatic. The movements become so well-rehearsed that they require progressively less attention. One can even begin to woolgather or think about what comes next, while the task runs off almost unconsciously, with less and less effort. At this point, we say that we finally have the particular skill "in our fingers" because that's just the way it feels.

Marc Anthony implored the Romans to "lend me your ears!" This metaphor was a request for the undivided attention of the entire brain; attention to a forthcoming verbal message. Yet he would not have been satisfied had his audience merely listened; he also wanted them to comprehend and to be persuaded. Metaphorical language betrays our naive concepts. We "put words into someone's mouth" rather than into someone's brain or mind. Common sense can obviously be misleading.

In the face of all this self-evident experience regarding the location of various skills, only some special theory would direct the search for language ability to a place where nobody actually felt it to be. Yet just such a theory existed in Europe in the year 1800. The totally discredited science of phrenology, which held that human talents and dispositions were not only dependent upon the functions of the brain, but might be inferred with precision from the external appearance of the skull, was sufficiently popular at the time to be interdicted by the government as dangerous to religion. The founder and leading exponent of phrenology, anatomist Franz Joseph Gall, was said to have a friend who was a verbal memory expert, and who coincidentally had large protruding eyes. This may have led Gall to locate language ability in the front of the brain, right below the eyes. In spite of its fanciful inaccuracies, phrenology was part of an intellectual climate in which human characteristics were being conceptually related to specific parts of the brain. Concurrently, a host of medical researchers were attempting to relate symptoms of nervous and mental disease to post-mortem autopsy findings.

The breakthrough came in 1840 when Marc Dax, and later Paul Broca in 1861, noticed that a specific area in the left half of the brain was damaged in patients who had suffered a type of paralytic stroke which also interfered with speech. All these patients had a right-sided paralysis prior to death. In striking contrast, patients with left-sided paralysis who showed post-mortem brain damage in the exact symmetrical area on the right half of the brain, had not experienced language difficulties as part of their paralytic strokes. Dax reported the finding first, and the history books give him priority thanks to the later efforts of his son to set the record straight. But the special area in the left side of the brain was named "Broca's area" for the man who rediscovered it. Broca was a well-known surgeon and anthropologist who published his findings; Dax was a modest and obscure physician who reported his discovery at a medical meeting, but never published it. To what extent either or both of them were influenced by the then fashionable phrenology is purely conjectural.

Later in the century, it was observed that damage to different parts of the left side of the brain produced different types of language problems. The farther forward the disease, the greater the problem with fluency; the farther back, the greater the problem with comprehension. The important thing is that these discoveries ushered in a century of study of the left side of the brain in patients like Clay, who developed language symptoms. The result is a growing understanding of the physical substrate of language, which we shall outline presently.

Before explaining the brain's language mechanisms, we must qualify the notion that a complex activity is simply "located" in a certain part of the body, brain or elsewhere. Left brain supremacy for language ability is not controversial, but finer details are harder to pin down. We use the word location only to pinpoint a particular area where damage will maximally interfere with the function in question. Several illustrations will make this clear. If a person is bitten on the foot by a rattlesnake he may become delirious and irrational. We understand the mechanism, that the poison is carried to the brain via the bloodstream, and we therefore *locate the effect* in the brain rather than in the foot. This can be proved by placing a tourniquet between the bite and the rest of the body, which prevents the poisoned blood from reaching the brain, and thereby prevents delirium.

Similarly, a person who is shot through the liver may bleed

internally, with a resultant drop in blood pressure, and un-consciousness. The mechanism here, is that the blood supply to certain brain areas which maintain consciousness is insufficient, and again, we can locate the effect in the brain rather than the liver. This too can be proved by administering a transfusion which maintains the blood flow to the brain, causing the patient to regain consciousness even before the liver injury is repaired.

As another example, we reject the common sense notion that a particular skill is "in the fingers" since it is not lost when the fingers are amputated. This is proved by the ability to carry out the appropriate movements as soon as artificial fingers are provided. By the same token, certain speech comprehension difficulties are instantly corrected by a hearing aid which amplifies incoming speech sounds; we therefore locate the problem in the ear. But no amount of amplification will render an unknown foreign language comprehensible; consequently we locate this problem in the brain rather than in the ear.

Thus, a specific language function is "in" a particular part of the brain in the same sense that the "motion mechanism" of an automobile is more "in the crankshaft" than "in the tires or spark plugs." A few malfunctioning plugs, or a flat tire, will disrupt but not prevent the motion of the car; a broken crankshaft however, will completely stop the car. To pursue the analogy, the motion of the car is also completely stopped when it runs out of gas or when the ignition is turned off. Why do we not say that the motion is *located* in the gas tank or the ignition key? Such a remark sounds foolish if we understand the mechanism of an internal combustion engine. An automobile which stops because of an empty gas tank or because the ignition is turned off has nothing wrong with its intrinsic movement mechanism. This is proved by filling the tank or turning on the ignition key—normal motion then recommences. When the mechanism of a complex behavior is understood we then stop talking about where that behavior is "located" in the system.

Complex activities such as speaking or walking require the

cooperation of widespread areas of the brain. Some of these areas are more critical than others, and their damage leads more predictably to interference with the complex behavior, even though the remainder of the system is preserved intact. To say that the complex behavior is therefore "located in" the critical area represents a form of magical thinking akin to that which leads to the execution of the courier who brings bad news. There are indeed areas in the nervous system which are so critical to a certain function as to be absolutely unexpendable. If nerves in the arms or legs are cut, the muscles which they control will die. But "Broca's area" is not one of these critical areas, nor are most of the other brain areas which have been implicated in the problem of aphasia. For example, following damage to Broca's area, a patient may have difficulty speaking at some times but not at others. It is therefore important to keep the fallacy of "location" in mind. If the ensuing description of the organization of the left brain's language mechanism is taken in this spirit, certain misconceptions will be avoided. For instance, one could not surgically excise the mental dictionary or any selected part of it, or locate and tinker with the syntactic mechanism.

Recall the hierarchical organization of the speech code— from sounds, to syllables, to meaningful units, to words, to phrases, to sentences, to connected discourse, and finally conversation. How does the brain implement this process? It's important to realize that only the sounds, and the muscular movements responsible for them, are observable. All the rest is inferred from the study of spoken language and from the effects of various disease states, with resultant scientific controversy. We have attempted a synthesis of the major current ideas.

At the root of the language process is the emotional need for communication with another individual. Man is a social animal and generally detests the feeling of loneliness. That is why hermits are so rare, and solitary confinement is such a profound form of torture. Humans seek each other out for companionship even when nothing else is forthcoming from the social contact. Language communication, which for most

of us means verbal intercourse, is one of the essential ingre-
dients of companionship. Silent communion with others is
emotionally compelling, and even pleasurable, as a respite
from the norm of social chatter; so is self-inflicted solitude.
But prolonged deprivation of verbal conversation, even when
all other physical and social needs are being satisfied, has
earned the appellation, "the silent treatment." When silence
becomes the social norm, it is clearly a form of self-sacrificial
mortification, as in the vows of silence taken by Trappist
monks.

Conventional wisdom has always taught that language
begins with the baby's first word; that everything prior to this
is meaningless babble, and that the preverbal infant's needs
are mainly vegetative. Nothing could be further from the
truth. The fate of infants whose physical needs are attended
to, but who are deprived of all other human contact, has been
documented. They tend to die, and if they do survive, they
are mentally defective. The utterance of the first word is not
the beginning, but rather the end of a long process of language and intellectual development. This process is intrin-
sically conversational, involving the senses of taste, smell,
sound, vision and touch—the multimedia preverbal world of
infant communication. For this reason we begin our description of the language mechanism with the most ancient part of
the nervous system—the so-called "feeling brain." This part
of the brain motivates all activities. It generates the emotional
need which underlies every communicative event.

A newborn infant is always gobbling, not just milk, but
nonverbal world knowledge. To highly verbal people it may
be of ultimate importance that the baby one day says "mama"
or "bottle." But the baby certainly has an intimate knowledge
of mama, bottle, and many other things long before these
phenomena are actually named, and the baby could deal with
them even if they were never named. The left side of the
brain is not mature enough in early infancy to even accomplish the mechanical repetition of word sounds, much
less to use them as labels for such complex human interactions as "mama" and "bottle." Nor is naming even necessary,

since the world of the infant is geared to nonverbal communication.

Earlier, we described how the right side of the brain is specialized for three-dimensional space; faces, emotion, and nonverbal environmental sounds such as music, or animal and mechanical noises. It has recently been discovered that the right half of the brain matures earlier than the left half, corresponding to the mode of infant communication. The ability to articulate sounds isn't achieved until later in the first year of life, but control over the eyes, which permits visual analysis of space, is mature by the age of four months. When the physical distance between baby and mother precludes smelling, tasting, and touching, the infant communicates mainly by looking. Thus, the observation that the first months of life are speechless is only half the story. The infant is not yet ready to perform verbally. When we focus upon the activities that the infant is performing, we discover that nonverbal knowledge of the physical world is being accumulated at a fantastic rate. This nonverbal knowledge is absolutely necessary before a verbal name can mean anything.

It isn't difficult to learn the vocabulary of a foreign language because the world in which it is spoken is very much like our own, and we take that for granted. Learning a foreign word for "cup" amounts to relabelling, or, as we now say, *recoding a concept* that is already very familiar.

To learn the construction, "the cup's handle," involves knowing what a handle is in general, knowing that a cup can have one, and knowing that a cup is still a cup without one. In short, proper use of the word cup presupposes knowledge of what it is used for. Then, you can talk about "drinking out of a cup," or "drinking a cup of tea," but not "drinking a teacup." We all experience lack of nonverbal knowledge when forced to learn technical terms in some completely alien human activity. If told that some strange instrument is a "wrelk," and that the part of it that turns is the "rell," there is no way of knowing whether the wrelk remains the same without the rell. Only observation of how these terms are used under different conditions permits one to deduce the rule.

This is precisely the predicament of every human infant. To meaningfully begin to name anything presupposes a tremendous amount of nonverbal information about its function in the real world. This general world knowledge is not confined to the left side of the brain, and a very important part of it is undoubtedly in the right half of the brain.

Language messages reach the brain via the senses, our only possible link with the world around us. The five familiar senses are vision, hearing, touch, smell, and taste. Most of us take them so much for granted that we don't realize we suffer from an embarrassment of riches. Let's simplify by sticking to vision, hearing, and touch.

Many people don't appreciate that they can "read" via each of these three senses. The word "book" in this sentence is visual. But if someone reads out the letters, "B O O K," we can read via the sense of hearing. And if the letters "B O O K" are embossed on a page, we can "read" with our eyes closed, via the sense of touch, as in Braille. The same letters, traced on the skin of our forearm by another person using a pointed instrument, can be "read" as well. (The letters must be large enough, but smaller letters can be read this way on the palm of the hand. The sharpest "tactile vision" is on the fingertips.)

These demonstrations show that the brain can tune into various senses to glean the same information. The three senses can roughly substitute for each other. These senses are the input channels to the language mechanism in the left side of the brain.

Language messages leave the brain via speech, gesture, facial expression, and handwriting. We tend to think of speech and handwriting as the primary external evidence of language, but American Sign Language of the deaf is a formal gestural system as complex as speech. Perhaps American Indian sign language is more familiar to some readers. This was the universal language among tribes of Plains Indians who couldn't understand each others' speech.

Note that every one of these methods for transmitting language messages requires the movement of muscles. We have previously illustrated that the word "book" could reach the left side of the brain and be understood via the three input channels of vision, hearing, and touch. These input channels can thus substitute for each other to a large extent in the reception of language messages. In analogous fashion, different groups of muscles can substitute for each other when language messages from the left side of the brain are to be transmitted to another person. Thus we can say, or spell aloud, the word "goodbye" by means of speech muscles— vocal cords, throat, lips, tongue and, of course, chest muscles to pump the required air out of the lungs. We can also write the word "goodbye" with our hand muscles, shoulder muscles (try writing movements with your elbow), leg muscles (try writing movements with your big toe, especially on wet sand at the beach), or neck muscles (try holding a pencil in your teeth). Some of these muscles have never been used for writing before, yet decent legibility can be achieved.

This demonstration shows that the language mechanism can utilize various muscles to transmit the same information, and muscles, like senses, can substitute for each other. Any muscle which can transmit a message that is comprehensible to another human being can serve as an output channel for language from the left side of the brain.

Man is an imitative animal and so are his simian ancestors. Universal delight in the ability of a chimpanzee to imitate human behavior obscures the depressing regularity with which people imitate each other. Youngsters see through this with disarming clarity. Hopelessly in the grip of an unwritten cultural program which, if successful, will rear them to be reasonable facsimiles of their parents, some of the more endearing epithets they hurl back and forth are "monkey see, monkey do" and "copycat!" From one point of view this is encouraging. It suggests that children basically respect originality. From another vantage point, it tells us something important about the way the brain is specialized for language development.

Newborn infants gurgle and coo a lot, and these tend to be vowel sounds. They do not have enough control over the muscles of the lips, tongue, jaws, and palate to articulate the speech sounds which we recognizes as consonants. The mouth has its hands full, so to speak, with the breathing, sucking, spitting, and swallowing activities of a newborn. Newborns sometimes do produce consonants; a perfect "p" sound may be articulated in the process of spitting out some disliked food, but the sound is coincidental to another action and is not produced for its own sake.

Roughly midway through the first year of life, the so-called "babbling period" begins. The coordinating mechanisms in the brain are now sufficiently mature to show what kind of speech sounds infants can produce when they feel like it. Strangely enough, the inventory of sounds that is displayed is much larger than what will be needed for the language eventually to be spoken. An English-speaking baby, for example, spontaneously articulates many more than the forty-odd sounds it will later need for the sound system of that language. Many of the sounds initially produced will be appropriate to languages the child will never hear.

Man's brain is literally "wired up" at birth to generate the sounds of all possible languages in the world. But, stated this way, the last sentence is somewhat grandiose, if not misleading. In other words, people can only speak languages if the sound systems for those languages are within the capabilities of their bodies. Nature doesn't know in what particular culture a particular brain will be reared, and consequently provides a phonetic palette which the baby will spontaneously babble, and from which the adults can select what is appropriate. It follows that at this stage, all babies in the world sound alike. The mechanism responsible for the babbling lies astride the output channels, close to the brain areas which control the speech muscles. It can be conceived as a built-in plan or program, like the perforated paper roll of a player piano, which issues sequences of instructions to the speech muscles to randomly produce all speech sounds. We shall call it an output program. There is a separate program for each output channel, corresponding to the muscles involved in speech, gesture, and writing, respectively.

An imitation game then begins, usually between mother and child, in which some of the sounds babbled by the baby get special adult attention. These are merely those gurgles and babbles which sound something like the parents' native language. The mother seizes on these and repeats them, perhaps improving on them just a bit. Babbling is often repetitive, and some of the earliest sounds turn out to be "mama" and "dada" which is very flattering to parents.

Even before the baby imitates its first word it may be imitating the intonation of sentences in the language it will eventually speak. These are the melodic contours; the prosody of declarations, questions, imperatives, and objections. When the parents are quiet, or absent, the baby gets additional practice by imitating itself. Regardless of whether the model is another person's speech or its own, each imitation is both felt and heard by the baby. Eventually, the sound pattern of the parents' native language crystallizes from the babbling, and sounds which are not destined for that particular language disappear. At this stage, babies in different countries begin to sound very different from each other.

The babbling baby is not only selecting the fixed inventory of basic sounds in its native language; it is also learning the rules for their combination. For instance, "mama" is acceptable, but "amam" won't pass muster. It doesn't take a baby long to realize that some combinations are gleefully repeated while others seem to fall upon deaf ears. At this repetitive stage the child doesn't know why some, but not other sound combinations elicit a conversational response from the parent and undoubtedly doesn't care why. The response is the only imporant thing: "Somebody out there loves me." The language mechanism is always fueled by the underlying emotional need to communicate with the parent or caregiver. But the adult, perhaps unconsciously, has a clear criterion for responding differentially to the stream of babble.

Some of the baby's spontaneously combined sounds are meaningful in the language, and when the baby happens upon these at random it is "speaking" and not just babbling. Such happy accidents deserve and receive a reward. The result is that a pattern in the brain is strengthened; the re-warded sounds occur more often and cease to be accidents. At this intermediate stage of the imitation game, audiotape recordings of the babbling baby lulling itself to sleep—so-called "crib talk"—sound like a parody of the speech which is to come, that is: occasional long monologues replete with the prosody of phrases and sentences, the latter sometimes recog-nizable as questions, orders, objections, manifestos, etc. An occasional word is identifiable, but the overall syllable sequence of these utterances isn't. The native language in-tended (English, French, Chinese) may be clear, but the words are not.

How can an imput, in this case the mother's nonrandom repetition of a chance syllable sequence, affect the spontane-ous random activity of the output program? Obviously, the infant must first recognize the particular sounds the mother chooses to get excited about. For example, the infant's brain must be able to distinguish the sounds of two consonants, "b" and "d," and the two vowels, "a" and "e," before it can begin to distinguish the spoken words, "bed," "bad," "dab," and "dad." In a few years, in order to read these words, "b" must look different from "d," and "a" from "e"." The sheer detec-tion of such differences must precede any decision about their meaning. So the brain requires an input analyzer, which it indeed possesses. This pattern-recognition mechanism lies astride the input channels, close to the brain areas which first receive incoming impulses from the ears, eyes, and skin.

There is a separate input analyzer for each of the senses. This separation prevents us from seeing sounds and hearing flashes of light. It also enables us to compare concurrent input patterns so we can detect errors. Many of our adult words, such as "friendship" and "loyalty," are abstract and divorced from particular sensation. During language acquisition, an object or event that is named verbally is simultaneously seen, touched, smelled, and perhaps tasted. The baby's under-standing of "milk" might fall apart if milk suddenly tasted like vodka, looked green, felt textured, or smelled like smoke.

The constellation of attributes which defines the true object requires independent analysis of these sensual qualities. Thus, the anatomical separation of the earliest stages of pattern recognition is an insurance policy which has biological significance for human survival. Later on we shall see that the incompleteness of this initial separation permits us to read.

Once the infant's input analyzer can successfully detect a particular sound sequence, parental reinforcement preserves the pattern as a model; a standard of comparison which, in order to be effective, must communicate with the output program. This communication may be a direct instruction to imitate the model sounds, and/or indirect, in the sense of monitoring and commenting upon the difference between the model and the most recent imitation produced. The latter process is called feedback of an error signal. It is an assessment of degree of discrepancy between what is produced and the desired result.

The stage is now set for one of the momentous events in intellectual development; the act of repetition. An input pattern will be transformed into an output pattern, accomplished only by a wet, living piece of brain tissue; a mesh, consisting of billions of nerve cells, which has already shown itself capable of producing the word to be repeated, albeit by accident. The repetition is a reasonable facsimile of the model, like the repetition of a word by a parrot. The voice is different than the original, the pronunciation is not quite accurate, but the match is close enough to call it a success.

Many natural and man-made systems possess imitative capability. The Grand Canyon, or a tunnel, will echo the shouted word "hello" rather faithfully. The image reflected back by a mirror is a faithful copy of the original object or person. The world is full of copying devices, and the brains of birds and babies are among them. But brains perform a rather fancy kind of copying that distinguish them from mere mimeograph machines. Even literal repetition, when performed by a living brain, involves fantastic abstraction, the mechanics of which are still subject to scientific speculation.

Most people are sufficiently familiar with common audiotape recorders or dictating machines to understand this point with the help of a brief science fiction fantasy.

Say the word "hello" into an audiotape recorder in three different moods: elated (a delighted shout); sleepy (with a yawn); and annoyed (through clenched teeth). Now play back the three renditions. Would you be astounded if each of the three inputs were reproduced in exactly the same polite, modulated voice? We'd be equally astounded by a mirror which always reflected a full-face image, whether the person confronting it were in full-face, in three-quarter view, or in profile. Now reverse the process. Suppose you repeat "hello" into the microphone three times, each time in exactly the same polite, modulated voice. When the three identical renditions are played back, would you be astounded if they sounded elated, sleepy, and annoyed, respectively? This sort of copying machine transforms the uniform input word into several variations which are still recognizable as the same word.

Our audiotape recorder seems to equate different versions of an input or output, recognizing a more general class to which the words all belong—each idiosyncratic rendition is but a particular instance. Thus, the gadget should no longer be called a copier, but rather a mechanism for classifying, categorizing, or abstracting.

This is precisely what the brain of an eighteen-month-old baby accomplishes when it begins to repeat the word "mama." The baby can recognize and repeat the word regardless of whether its mother uttered the word when excited, relaxed, tired, amused, sad, or frightened. Each of these emotional states yields a physically different sound pattern of the word. Nevertheless, the baby can still recognize it, as well as recognize the word "mama" when spoken by a young sibling whose voice has a higher pitch than the mother's voice in any of her emotional states. The baby can also recognize the word when spoken by the father, although his voice is deeper than the mother's.

Repetition by a living brain is an active process. It involves analysis of the input, an unconscious decision process in which input patterns are classified into categories which are transformationally equivalent, and then a similarly abstract synthesis of output patterns. Viewing oneself on closed circuit television in the supermarket, or playing back a recording of one's own voice is intermediate between the active way the brain "copies," and the passive world of echoes and mirror images. TV systems and audiotape recorders actually analyze the input pattern and resynthesize it to produce the output or playback. However, the connection between analysis and resynthesis is passive and slavish. No concept intervenes; what goes in, comes out.

An imitative mechanism must therefore be included in the developing concept of the overall language system. It should be stressed, however, that this mechanism contains the active categorizing capability just described. Understanding of this sophisticated capability is required to do justice to current psychological understanding of the imitative process. It also gives us the freedom to make fascinating mistakes, such as mishearing a word or saying something incorrectly. Once the intervening process between input and output patterns is active, rather than passive and slavish, other influences in the brain can affect it, with resultant human frailty. In contrast, ordinary mirrors and voice recorders don't lie; they show things as they are, but not as they might be.

Lest the abstract quality of simple imitation seem too glorified, we hasten to add that all the transformations involved are low-level ones. The dimension of complexity is illustrated by a typographical transformation used repeatedly on this page—capitalization. The shift key on a typewriter permits any letter to be typed in either lower or upper case. But the complexity of the change varies from letter to letter. In the following, the change is mainly one of scale, or of some non-critical detail which preserves the shape of the letter:

c,f,k,o,p,s,u,v,w,x,y,z
C,F,K,O,P,S,U,V,W,X,Y,Z

In contrast, the transformation between upper and lower case in the following example entails a comparatively gross recoding of the letter's shape:

$$b,d,g,h,n,q,r$$
$$B,D,G,H,N,Q,R$$

Physical similarity breaks down more drastically in the latter group of letters, so there is less opportunity to accomplish the transformation by sheer matching of shapes. It is necessary to know a specific rule for each letter, that R means r for example. This higher level of complexity in the transformation is getting beyond the imitative capability of the un-comprehending repetition mechanism. If we wrote the letter X on a page, a young child might copy it as the smaller version x without even realizing that it was part of the alphabet. But one would be astounded if, in the same state of ignorance, the child copied R as r.

The case of verbal copying is completely analogous. A baby trying to imitate the word "dog" may approximate it by varied pronunciations such as "dug," "doog," or "dud," but an attempted repetition that sounded like "chien," "spaniel," or "setter" would be disconcerting if it came from a brain that did not yet know the meaning of the word "dog."

The point to note about the imitation mechanism is that it needn't comprehend the meaning of the pattern being copied. We can repeat speech in a foreign language without under-standing it, or copy mathematical equations that are mean-ingless to us. Opera singers can learn a role phonetically. Al-though imitation is the most basic language skill, it can be "mindless." The quality which makes it meaningful is at-tributable to the syntactic-semantic mechanism. In a nutshell, it is this ability which enables us to paraphrase a sentence or to actually carry out instructions. Although the imitative mechanism develops prior to the syntactic-semantic mecha-nism, after the latter matures both function together as a unit. Their separability, and the further subdivision of syntactic and semantic mechanisms, only surfaces when normal communication breaks down. A few examples will make this clear.

Question: "Do you have a match?"

Answer No. 1: "Do you have a match?"
Answer No. 2: "Do I have a match?"
Answer No. 3: "Sorry, I don't."

Question: "What is your name?"

Answer No. 1: "What is your name?"
Answer No. 2: "What is my name?"
Answer No. 3: "Fred."

Note that in each example, the first answer is an exact repetition of the words in the question; in fact, the answer might be an echo. The second answer in each example is an appropriate grammatical transformation of the question. Syntactical understanding is in evidence. However, the purpose of the question was missed. The third answer in each example indicates an understanding of the question and an appropriate semantic response. There is an appreciation of the intent of the question.

These illustrations suggest that the syntactic-semantic mechanism develops through the superimposition of social awareness upon rote repetition. The basic problem is the separation between "I" and "thou." The first answer to each question misses this distinction. The second answer acknowledges the distinction between the questioner and answerer, but misses the point of the question. The third answer seems to apprehend the intent in the mind of the questioner.

People can understand many things they would never say; language comprehension always outstrips language production. The same is true at the earliest stages of language acquisition. The infant understands verbal statements long before speaking them, but this is difficult to prove conclusively. If comprehension seems to occur, the objection can always be raised that the baby is responding to cues from the whole situational context of the sentence, or to nonverbal cues from the tone of voice, or facial expression of the speaker. Unfortunately, babies do not converse with people who are outside of their field of vision so the crucial experiments are difficult to perform. For this reason, the activity of the syntactic-semantic mechanism cannot be demonstrated prior to the onset of speech in the second year of life. This usually begins with one-word "sentences" in which the baby points to a seen object and names it, demonstrating the beginning of the semantic function.

The syntactic function begins to appear with the advent of two-word "sentences," such as "Jimmy hungry," Jimmy sleepy," "more milk," or "more cookie." The grammar develops very rapidly from that time on, and ingenious experiments can prove that the child always understands constructions which are more complex than the ones being produced spontaneously.

The physical "location" of the syntactic-semantic mechanism becomes crystallized by adulthood. The critical area for interfering with these functions adjoins the site in the left half of the brain where the auditory input is analyzed.

The reason for distinguishing syntactic from semantic mechanisms is that brain lesions which produce aphasia indicate that these mechanisms are indeed separable. This will be explained further in Chapter Six which deals with language breakdown. For the present, it is regrettable that less is known about the possible brain mechanisms underlying this central language function than all the others discussed. Theories exist which propose conceivable brain mechanisms for the imitation game in all its abstract complexity. However, a brain mechanism for transformation of present to past tense has never been imagined.

This completes our sketch of the neurology of language as presently conceived. Each of the levels of the linguistic process described in the previous chapters has intelligible neurological reality (see also the diagram in Chapter 6, page 134).

We must inquire about the origin of the language ability of the left side of the brain. Is it there at birth, or is it taught to

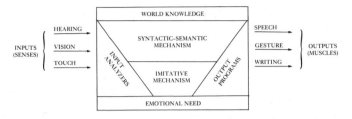

A diagrammatic summary of the major language mechanisms which account for the development and maintenance of human communication.

children by their parents? Ever since people began to wonder whether language was of divine origin or a human invention there have been two schools of thought on the subject. At one extreme are those who argue that language ability is inborn and simply unfolds on its own when the child reaches a certain age—just the way the child begins to crawl and walk when it is ready. This is one of the oldest notions in recorded history, and one of its earliest appearances can be found in Herodotus:

Herodotus, the Greek historian (484–420 B.C.), describes "how the Egyptians, before the reign of Psammitichus, considered themselves to be the most ancient of mankind. But afterward Psammitichus, having come to the throne, endeavoured to ascertain who were the most ancient. From the time they considered the Phrygians to have been before them, and themselves before all others. Now, when Psammitichus was unable, by inquiry, to discover any solution of this question, who were the most ancient of men, he devised the following expedient: He gave two new-born children of poor parents to a shepherd, to be brought up among his flocks in the following manner: he gave strict orders that no one should utter a word in their presence, that they should lie in a solitary room by themselves, and that he should bring goats to them at certain times, and that when he had satisfied them with milk he should attend to his other employments. Psammitichus contrived and ordered this, for the purpose of hearing what word the children would first articulate after they have given over their insignificant mewlings; and such accordingly was the result. For when the shepherd had pursued this plan for the space of two years, one day as he opened the door and went in, both the children falling upon him, and holding out their hands, cried "Becos." The shepherd when he first heard it said nothing; but when this same word was constantly repeated to him whenever he went and tended the children, he acquainted his master. By his command he brought the children into his presence. When Psammitichus heard the same, he enquired what people called anything by name "Becos" and discovered that the Phrygians called bread by that name. Thus the Egyptians, convinced, allowed that the Phrygians were more ancient than they. I had this from the priests of Vulcan at the temple of Memphis." [3]

At the other extreme are those who believe that the mind of a newborn babe is like a blank slate and that all language is learned. They argue that childrearing practices in every culture are geared to turning out reasonable facsimiles of adults' behavior patterns. Children imitate their elders in language as in other customs.

The debate in this naive form is now considered a "straw man." It turns out that both positions are right, and therefore both are partially wrong. Recent research shows that the brain of a newborn infant comes already equipped with built-in speech ability which seems to be more in the left side of the brain than in the right. We can demonstrate this by making speech sounds such as "ba," "ga," or "da" while we record the brain waves from the infant's skull. The waves recorded from the left side of the head are more "turned on" by these speech sounds than waves recorded from the right side of the head. The situation is just the reverse when nonverbal sounds, such as musical tones, are played to the baby. Also, at about the age of six months, all babies in the world began to babble in the same way, regardless of their environments. We have described this babbling as containing all the potential sounds of the world's languages. If this is the true onset of speech, another point is scored for those who believe language to be innate.

We then described how the spontaneous babbling was sys-

3. Herodotus, *The Histories*, Bk. II.

tematically edited by the adult caregiver to mold the sound system of the native tongue. Doesn't this show that language is learned by imitation rather than being inborn? Even if there are some innate babbling mechanisms to provide raw materials for adults to work with, doesn't the social environment then take over the whole operation? After all, a Chinese baby adopted at birth by an English-speaking family will be speaking perfect English a few years later, and will have no comprehension of Chinese.

Still, there are curious jumps in language development which don't seem to have anything to do with imitation in a simple sense. For example, here's a two-year-old who only speaks single words such as "milk," "truck," and "cookie." While eating lunch one day, having finished her milk and cookie, she demands seconds by simply shouting "milk! cookie!." These were indeed available, but her ambitious mother felt the moment ripe for creation. Rather than capitulate abjectly and serve up seconds on command, her mother kept repeating "more milk, more cookie" after each single word demand. This went on for a while until the child said "more milk, more cookie" and was instantly rewarded with seconds. But more importantly, the child was also rewarded with the image of an exultant mother. That very evening, when the child was dallying with her truck at bedtime, the toy was taken away from her. To her parents' amazement, she shouted "more truck," a statement she had never heard from them since they didn't speak that way. The child had grasped a grammatical principle—"more anything." This principle was spontaneously applied to create a new utterance which could not have been an imitation.

As a second example, another child of the same age spoke present-tense "sentences" exclusively; for example, "Daddy go bye-bye" and "Daddy fix the car." One fine day he imitated the past tense, "Daddy fixed the car." The next day, after his father had left the house, he spontaneously said, "Daddy go-ed bye-bye." Again, this was a grammatical construction he had never actually heard because his parents would never say it that way. Those who hold that language ability is primarily innate relish such observations. These examples, they argue, furnish powerful evidence that basic language skills are not simply learned by imitation. It appears that children can deduce abstract grammatical principles, such as qualification of nouns by adverbs, and the suffix rule for the past tense of regular verbs, all on their own. This is proved by the fact that the child spontaneously applies these rules creatively, if incorrectly, to novel situations which cannot possibly be imitations of adult speech. Thus, they argue, this mysteriously language ability must be an innate capacity of the brain.

There is merit in both arguments. Both nature and nurture—heredity and environment—contribute to language development. The scientist's job is to assess the balance of their relative contributions. This is no idle academic exercise but rather a question which affects the future health and pocketbook of every citizen. If language is primarily inborn, we tend to treat its disorders by modifying the brain, using drugs and surgery; if it is primarily environmental, we tend to treat its disorders by educational methods. To make matters even more complicated, the balance of nature-nurture factors may vary in different types of communication disorders.

Let's now restate our original question: "What is the origin of the language ability of the left side of the brain?" The answer is that it is inborn, part of the genetic endowment of the human race. However, like a seed which will never become a plant in the absence of a favorable environment of soil, water, and sunlight, the innate language mechanism has certain critical requirements. These must be met if an intelligent human personality is to develop. The requirements are threefold: 1) at least one route for language messages to get into the brain; 2) at least one route for language messages to get out of the brain; and 3) an appropriate environment, consisting of at least one other adaptable human being.

Thus, the language mechanism is innate, but it requires human conversation for its development.

6

Communication
Breakdown

How does aphasia fit into the last two chapters? This type of question is asked by most students in the freshman and sophomore years (the so-called "preclinical" years) of medical school. They expect to become doctors and therefore expect to study disease. Instead, they are first subjected to intensive training in the structure and function of the *normal* human body. The breakdown of any system can only be understood in terms of its healthy state. Think about it. We'd certainly mistrust an automobile mechanic who wasn't well-versed in the structure and function of a smoothly running internal combustion engine. Similarly, a demystified explanation of aphasia requires some technical knowledge of what language is in the first place, and how the nervous system is organized to make use of it.

Let's see how communication breaks down. What are the effects of damage to the system we have built up so laboriously? Recall that each component which we have labeled corresponds to some important aspect of the communication process. There is no necessary reason for a stroke to selectively damage any particular function. As a matter of fact, such selective damage is the exception rather than the rule.

But the occasional loss of one specific facet of the communication process is probably the reason for our noticing its separate existence in the first place.

The most important principle to realize is that damage to *any part* of the system can cause a severe communication disorder. But as we shall see in a moment, only some of these disorders are called "aphasia." Indeed, the more we understand about the way the system works, the less we tend to label a given disorder "aphasia." Perhaps this is the solution to the great mystery which we described previously, that the peculiar linguistic specialization of the left side of the brain was not discovered until the nineteenth century. Since all communication disorders share common features, the very special ones which we now call aphasia could easily have gotten lost in the shuffle. The following are a list of specific communication disorders associated with various parts of the system.

Emotional need (damage to the "feeling brain"): At the root of every communicative act is the emotional desire to engage in it, therefore, severe damage to this part of the mechanism plays havoc with the biological purpose of language itself. The patient may have speech but not seem to use it, or the distorted balance of impulses of sexuality, fear, and rage may render communication delirious, with severe alterations of memory and consciousness. Language remains, but becomes irrelevant to communication. Fortunately, these conditions are an extremely rare effect of stroke.

World knowledge: Our links to the present are simple and basic. There is awareness of who one is; where one is presently located (home, street, city, state, country); calendar and clock time (year, month, date, time of day); identity of one's conversational partner (friend, relative, stranger, nurse, doctor); one's probable present situation (sick, well, confused, on vacation, at work, hospitalized); and one's relation to others (being helped, being cared for, being exploited, etc.). If these links to current reality are broken, the patient is said to be *disoriented* but not aphasic. The language mechanism functions properly but the loss of world knowledge is such as to render it irrelevant to ongoing communication.

The normal process of aging makes breakdown of this part of the mechanism familiar. Memory of recent events fails, but since the remainder of the language machinery is unaffected, communication simply becomes progressively more irrelevant to current events. For example, the mechanics of conversation proceed normally, but the patient seems to dwell increasingly on the past. The earliest phases merge into the normal tendency of the aged to self-preoccupation and reminiscence; at its best this represents a summing up, a historical perspective, and perhaps even wisdom, if others can learn from it. But, if links with the present are broken, and past becomes the present, dementia has begun.

Input channels: The most common disorders of the input channels to an otherwise normal brain are deafness and blindness. An eye or an ear has but a single nerve leading from it to its respective analyzer in the brain. This highly vulnerable channel is easily interrupted. By comparison, the skin surface covers the whole body. We have no real counterpart, in touch sensation, for the phenomenon of total blindness or deafness in an otherwise healthy individual. That is, people can be totally blind or deaf or both, but total loss of touch sensation is virtually impossible. We have seen that each of these three senses can serve as an adequate input channel to the language mechanism in the left side of the brain. Helen Keller's triumph over both blindness and deafness, with touch being the only point of contact between her innate language capacity and other people's messages, thereby becomes intelligible, if no less miraculous. In her adult life, she was able to understand speech by holding her fingertips lightly against the speaker's lips.

It might seem almost a matter of indifference whether vision, hearing, or touch is used as an input channel for language. For the normal adult, capable of learning Braille and sign language, and forced to choose among vision, hearing, and touch as a sole remaining input channel, there would certainly be esthetic preferences. But the situation is very different if the input channel is lost prior to speech development. A person who is blind at birth, but who has normal hearing, can learn to speak eloquently. But a sighted person who is deaf from infancy will rarely learn to speak normally. Apparently, the child must actually hear both his own and his parents' speech in the original imitation game to fully realize the innate capacity to transmit verbal messages.

We have seen that the language mechanism is extremely adaptable to varying output channels, provided the messages they transmit are intelligible to others. Thus, the deaf child who is trained to be proficient in sign language and lip-reading, can develop a normal language mechanism in spite of the speech deficiency. These children achieve gratifying human communication, literacy, occupational competence, and occasionally, intellectual brilliance and artistic creativity.

What happens if all input channels are cut off? As noted before, this is almost impossible to accomplish, but the question is sufficiently intriguing to scientists that they have tried to answer it experimentally. These are called "sensory deprivation" experiments. If a person is floating face down in water, suitably attired in a diving mask for breathing purposes, he is weightless. Stimulation by gravity ceases. With blindfold and earplugs, light and sound stimulation are prevented. Proper packing of the arms and legs in soft material within rigid encasing tubes makes it difficult to achieve sensation by means of touch or movement of joints. The water is kept at body temperature so there is no sensation of cold or warmth. It is the ultimate in solitary confinement. The environment is "locked out." Volunteers for these experiments tend to hallucinate an environment which they cannot experience directly.

Output channels: Just as we distinguished localized disorders of input channels, we must now distinguish localized disorders of output channels. These disorders interfere with the flow of language messages to muscles which execute the messages, or interfere with the muscles themselves. Obviously, paralysis or removal of the vocal cords or tongue will interfere with speech output, but not with writing. Nor does paralysis or amputation of the right hand preclude writing with the left hand. As with the disorders of input channels, the communication problems resulting from disorder of one output channel can be overcome by substituting another.

What would happen to a person deprived of all output channels? We don't really know, but there is one neurological condition which comes close to total output deprivation. It is known as the "locked-in" syndrome and is fortunately a rare consequence of stroke; only a handful of cases have ever been described. This condition results from localized brain damage which spares the language mechanism as well as the input channels for vision and hearing. However, there is a bottleneck of output channels in the affected area, and speech muscles and all limb and facial muscles are paralyzed, with the sole exception of the muscles that move the eyes. Such patients give no evidence of being able to communicate via language, but their eye movements follow the examiner, so they appear to be alert. Several perceptive neurologists have noticed the following: if the patient is told that moving the eyes *up* means "yes" and moving the eyes down means "no," he could then reply intelligently to any question requiring a simple "yes" or "no" answer.

The problem is how to converse with somebody who possesses a two-word vocabulary. With ingenuity this has been accomplished, and it became clear that the patient comprehended everything normally. Using a questioning format familiar from popular TV shows such as "What's My Line?" or the game of Twenty Questions, the examiner frames questions which can honestly be answered affirmatively or negatively. To discover a thought in the mind of a person with a "yes-no" vocabulary, it is only necessary that he or she comprehend questions, and answer them truthfully. This "locked-in" state illustrated the adaptability of an intact language mechanism in the face of impoverished output channels. It also points out the extent to which conversational ingenuity can help to overcome a communication disorder. At last report, one such patient was directing his family's affairs by means of this two-word vocabulary.[4]

Input analyzers: Recall that each input channel in our diagram was said to have a separate analyzer that physically oc-

4. Of course, such patients could learn Morse code, using "eyes up" for a dot and "eyes down" for a dash. They could then communicate spontaneously albeit slowly, to somebody who knew that code.

cupied a separate area on the brain's surface. In these regions, preliminary analyses of incoming messages occurs. Since these regions share the same brain, they are not as widely separated as their respective input channels—the eyes, ears, and fingertips. Yet they are sufficiently separated so that each can be individually affected by a stroke in different areas of the brain.

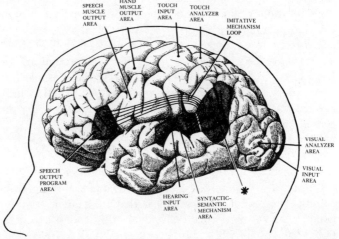

The darkened areas show the primary language centers of the left side of the brain which are implicated in aphasia. Learning to read involves the association of a *visual* pattern with a *touchable* object that already has an *acoustic* name. The star (*) marks an area unique to man which interrelates the analyzers for these three senses (vision, hearing, and touch). It is presumed to be important for reading skills. (Adapted from "Language and the Brain" by N. Geschwind. Copyright © April, 1972 by Scientific American Inc., p. 78. All rights reserved.)

Direct damage to one of the analyzers, or its disconnection from other mechanisms in the diagram, produces bizarre communication disorders that affect only one sense, leaving others intact.

If only the visual analyzer is affected, the patient may be able to see, but may not be able to crystallize the exact pattern seen. This would render the visual world highly unreliable, including the printed page. Embossed letters could still be read via the sense of touch, and spoken messages would be perfectly intelligible. The problem in reading would merely be part of a general problem of seeing shapes. However, if this analyzer is not damaged but simply disconnected from the syntactic-semantic mechanism, words become just a meaningless pattern printed on paper, like a foreign language. This disorder is called "word blindness," and it means that the word can be seen clearly but cannot be recognized as written speech. Such patients may still be able to express their thoughts in writing; the syntactic-semantic mechanism remains connected to the output apparatus. Yet, they cannot read what they have written.

If only the auditory analyzer is affected, the patient may be able to hear sound, but may not be able to resolve the precise pattern that permits its identification. Thus, the crumpling of paper may be indistinguishable from speech, and words like "pit, bit, wit, sit," may all sound the same. The world of sound would become highly unreliable as input, even though reading ability would be undisturbed. Here, the problem of comprehending speech is merely part of a general problem of distinguishing sound patterns. However, if this analyzer is not damaged, but only disconnected from the syntactic-semantic mechanism, words, though clearly heard, become meaningless sound patterns again like a foreign language. This disorder is called "word deafness." Spontaneous speech is unaffected in these patients because the syntactic-semantic mechanism remains connected to the output apparatus. However, if their speech is tape-recorded and played back to them, they cannot understand what they have said.

Output programs: Each output channel in our diagram was said to have its own program, one that physically occupies a separate area on the brain's surface. This enables the syntactic-semantic mechanism to select from a variety of output channels (muscle groups). Thus, discrete damage, or disconnection of any particular program, can disorganize verbal expression via a single route, leaving others intact. For example, a patient may have trouble writing words he can both say and spell aloud, or vice versa, as in the case of Samuel Johnson. Clay's illness illustrates this principle: he was unable to write or type the manuscript for this book intelligibly enough for it to be read by anyone else, but he was able to dictate it into a tape recorder, roughly as it appeared in Chapters One and Two.

In contrast to the input analyzers which are spread over widely dispersed regions of the brain, the main output programs for speech and writing movements are relatively bunched together in the front part of the left brain. This renders them particularly vulnerable to joint disruption. It is much more likely that a single injury will damage them en masse, rather than individually. This is illustrated by the following case history.

An educated, sophisticated writer has had a stroke. He fears that his intellect has suffered since he finds it difficult to speak his thoughts well enough to be understood. This seems surprising since he understands everything that is said to him, as well as programs on television. As his speech slowly recovers he asks for reading materials. To his delight, he can understand newspaper and magazine stories. Writing materials are then called for. To his consternation, his writing ability is as disorganized as his partially recovered speech. What is most curious is that the muscles used for writing and speaking are not paralyzed. He muses:

At the age of five I could converse fluently—that is, both understand and produce speech. Then I went to school where I learned to read and write. Fifty years later a stroke bombed me back to infancy. During recovery, I became aware of great difficulty in expressing my thoughts in speech. I felt my intellectual development had been reversed. Naturally, I expected to lose my formal education—reading and writing—rather than the speaking skills which had been mastered in preschool years. I also expected my recovery to retrace the chronological sequence of my intellectual development, like growing up all over again. That is, my speech should have recovered first so that I could engage in ordinary conversations. Following this, the later skills—reading and writing—should have been recovered.

To my amazement, it didn't work like that at all. At the very beginning of my recovery I could already read and listen, with almost complete comprehension. Yet, even months later, my speech and writing are still a mess. Why don't reading and writing go together as they did in elementary school? Why is reading grouped with listening, and both skills unimpaired, whereas writing is grouped with speaking, and these are both still rough and primitive?

Massive damage to his output program areas have interfered with this patient's powers of verbal expression. He can't blame the difficulty on paralyzed muscles of the hand or mouth—these muscles are well under his control as long as he doesn't try to use them for speaking or writing. It seems as if these muscles had lost contact with the idea of verbal expression—had been disconnected from the imitative and syntactic-semantic mechanisms. The mental concepts cannot get through to these muscles, just as a tennis serve or golf stroke gets "rusty." But the patient has retained powers of verbal comprehension—listening and reading. All his inputs, their respective analyzers, and his syntactic-semantic mechanisms remain in good shape and are properly connected.

The point is that intellect doesn't fall apart according to the way it was put together. The childhood progression of acquiring particular skills (for example speech and verbal comprehension before reading and writing), does not seem to matter. The important thing is their spatial organization in the brain.

This type of case is the first form of "aphasia" that was clearly described in the nineteenth century. In the intervening years, many experts have felt that the term "aphasia" should be reserved for damage to the syntactic-semantic mechanism—which remains intact in these patients. The terminology is really unimportant. What is important is that the undeniable tragedy of demolished expressive skills is somehow mitigated by the preservation of verbal comprehension.

How do such patients cope with the damage to the output program? Their major problem is the loss of verbal fluency. They speak and write slowly and with great effort, as if to

force planned sentences through a bottleneck in their conversion to sound or graphic patterns. The typical strategy
adopted is one we have described in Chapter four, that of
telegrammatic speech. Only the accented, stressed, informa-
tion-bearing words of sentences are uttered; the unaccented,
unstressed, function words—the articles, conjunctions, prepositions, and pronouns—tend to be deleted. An example
follows:[5]

Question: "Where is your daughter?"

Answer: "New Orleans . . . home . . . Monday."

Question: "Will she stay home?"

Answer: "No . . . no . . . bridesmaid . . . working . . . married
. . . no"

Such a patient would have trouble repeating an expression
such as, "No ifs, ands, or buts," which consists completely of
words that the telegrammatic strategy tends to omit.

Despite the fluency difficulty, even a severe disorder of the
output programs rarely interferes with meaningful communication. The patient's auditory comprehension is intact,
but this is a mixed blessing. He can understand the speech of
others, but unfortunately he can also understand his own.
Since speech output is so inferior to the intended utterance,
self-consciousness of performance occurs, a frustrating, de-
moralizing, and depressing experience.

It may be instructive to compare the effect of this type of
damage in the case of a highly literate deaf-mute who normally communicates in both the American Sign Language of
the deaf and written English. What happens when such a per-

5. In this and the next chapter, quotes from patients other than Clay are
taken from J. M. Wepman and L. V. Jones, "Five Aphasias: A Commentary
on Aphasia as a Regressive Linguistic Phenomenon," in D. McK. Rioch and
E. A. Weinstein, eds., *Disorders of Communication: Proceedings of the Association
for Research in Nervous and Mental Disease*, 42 (Baltimore: Williams & Wilkins,
1964), pp. 190–203. Our interpretations of the protocols differ somewhat.

son experiences a stroke which widely damages the output programs but leaves all input and syntactic-semantic mechanisms intact? These cases are rare, and can only be evaulated by professionals who understand sign language, an even rarer combination.

Prior to her stroke, a patient, deaf from birth, could converse fluently with anyone who knew sign language, by means of the gestural output channel. She had also learned to read, write, and type in English, as a "second language." Following the same type of stroke as the previous patient, her signing, writing, and typing were hard to decipher. But she could still comprehend sign language produced by others, and could still understand English text. The principle illustrated here once again is that speech and language are not synonymous. Speech is merely the most common code for transmitting language.

Imitation mechanism: Recall that the "copycat" skill is one of the earliest to mature in the first year of life. It is a basic talent of the brain that we share with monkeys, apes, and parrots. This shouldn't be surprising inasmuch as we are social animals who are born in an immature state. Each of us is then shaped by our parents into the people we eventually become. To accomplish this feat in the short span of a few years, we had best be talented imitators.

Occasionally, a stroke may primarily damage the imitative machinery, leaving the remainder of the language mechanism relatively intact. The following case history illustrates this.

This particular patient sustained a common form of stroke, one that hardly interfered with his ability to participate in spoken conversation. He seemed to understand most of what was said to him, and his remarks were reasonably intelligible, although the sounds he produced were a bit garbled. However, the examination turned up a curious symptom which might escape casual observation.

Most of us would agree that it unusual for a participant in ordinary adult social conversation to request an exact repetition of something said. Nevertheless, the examination of patients with brain damage routinely includes instructions to repeat the examiner's comments verbatim. This procedure occasionally leads to astounding observations. In the present case, it was noticed that in spite of his ability to converse relatively well, the patient could not repeat the examiner's sentences verbatim. He could paraphrase the sentence verbally, which indicated he had indeed understood it. He could carry out the actions that the sentence indicated, such as "Shut the door," or "May I have a match?" which also proved that they were comprehended. But, literal repetition of the sentence was relatively difficult. This is a curious inversion of the pattern to be expected from a very young child who can easily repeat words and sentences that he or she cannot possibly understand. Cases of this type constitute additional evidence that the imitative mechanism is somewhat separable from the rest of the language apparatus, even in adulthood. The imitative mechanism copies without comprehension; the semantic-syntactic mechanism comprehends but cannot imitate.

Why was the patient's spontaneous speech a bit garbled? This isn't supposed to happen if the syntactic-semantic mechanism and the output programs are both intact and connected. Apparently, the imitative mechanism does double duty in adulthood, and is not as autonomous as our diagrams or the examiner's tests might suggest. In the midst of natural conversation, the brain works as a whole. That's why it takes very specialized types of examinations to demonstrate the underlying mechanisms.

Syntactic-semantic mechanism: This is the heart of the language mechanism—responsible for the so-called "deep structure" of the grammar of language. There are purists who contend that only brain damage of this type deserves to be called "aphasia." They argue that the effects of damage to input, output, or imitative components of the language mechanism can all be circumvented with ingenuity; even gross deficit of world knowledge, as seen in senility and mental retardation, is compatible with functional communication at some level. They have a point. Semantic and syntactic operations are certainly critical for the understanding and production of most of what we mean by "language." Let us begin to describe their breakdown with one of the most dramatic cases in neurological history.

This patient did not have a stroke. She was found in a coma following a suicide attempt by gas. On recovering consciousness, she could not converse. She never again spoke intelligible sentences spontaneously, nor did she give evidence of understanding remarks made by others. She had also lost the ability to read and write. However, she did repeat what she heard verbatim, like an "echo box." This repetition was apparently accomplished without comprehension. The principle illustrated is verifiable in everyone's experience: "echoing" or "parroting" of speech is a fundamental capability of the brain. It does not require that the repeated remark be understood. Post-mortem examination of this woman's brain revealed an unprecedented partition of the language mechanism, attributable to the special way in which the gas affected the brain's circulation. Input and output channels, their analyzers and programs, and the connecting imitative mechanism were undisturbed. This machinery was sufficient to support her rote repetition ability. But this intact section of brain was disconnected from the remainder of the language apparatus, most notably from the semantic-syntactic mechanism. Thus, she could "echo" a command but neither paraphrase nor comply with it. The latter two actions would, of course, entail the analysis of the meaning of the command.

More commonly, a stroke produces less drastic damage which only partially interferes with the semantic-syntactic mechanism. Remember that our ability to understand telegrams and headlines divides vocabulary into two broad categories. The content words carry the burden of meaning (the semantic load)—they define what we are talking about. The function words act as connective glue to show the relationship among the content words. We have previously seen that damage to the output program creates a loss in fluency. Speech tends to be so effortful that function words are often omitted without severe loss to communication. They are omitted but clearly implied, and we "get the message" just as we do with telegrams and newspaper headlines.

With injury to the semantic-syntactic component fluency is retained. But there is sometimes a much more alarming loss, namely, the tendency to omit substantive content words. This leads to a vacuous fluency, with vocabulary limited to the more frequent words of the language. In the following example, a patient was asked about her family, and responded:

Yes! . . . when I know. If I know that they're good, they're wonderful. Why don't I say what we have, because we have everything. But good, they're good. They are good to me.

Note the failure of explicit communication. The grammatical form of phrases and sentences is retained, as is fluency, rhythm, and melody of speech. However, the paucity of substantive content words renders the description vague, general, and primarily emotional.

This aphasic problem is largely *semantic*. The patient knows what she means but usually cannot generate the unique word, *le mot juste*, that clinches the intention of the sentence. Once the deficient semantic content is supplied, in the examiner's questions, verbal comprehension is immediately demonstrated. In milder cases, or during recovery, this form of the disorder seems like an everyday type of forgetfulness in which names of things are lost. Nouns are, of course, all fairly infrequent words. If they can't be recalled, their meaning can still be conveyed by circumlocution; for example, "Please pass me the . . . you know, the red stuff in the bottle that you pour on a hamburger." Syntactic skills are normal, and this form of aphasia is the converse of the telegrammatic pattern which results from damage to the output programs.

A second form of damage to the semantic-syntactic component seems to affect the *syntactic* mechanism at its very heart, interfering with the organization of sentences, phrases, and occasionally, of words, even though the semantic content is freely available. This is illustrated in the next example, by a patient who is attempting to describe a picture. The picture shows a living room scene with a man in the foreground and a woman entering from the rear.

Here's a home . . . nice home . . . former a treasure . . . a like that each here . . . ace steward . . . and a book he's aiding . . . and floor lamps and every book . . . look at the picturer . . . sokd on has aird . . . he has a them.

Although both function *and* content words appear, there is a noticeable relaxation of syntactic constraint; that is, word order seems at times to be randomly scrambled. Inappropriate content words are semantically related to the intended word. The net result is that it's not exactly clear what the patient is trying to communicate, even though we know the picture that constitutes the subject matter. In the absence of the picture, in natural conversation or perhaps on the telephone, the message would be even more cryptic.

As might be expected with such a critical defect of syntactic function, the patient's comprehension of written or spoken utterances is usually severely disturbed. Self-awareness is also impaired. The patient is seemingly blissfully oblivious to the fact that he or she is not making sense to others. This uncritical attitude has been used to explain a rather bizarre symptom—the frequent euphoric mood of these patients. By any ordinary human reckoning they'd be expected to be distressed and frustrated. Nevertheless, they may not only deny that they are sick and hospitalized, but that anything is wrong with their speech.

How does such a patient come to grips with the glaring failure of his conversations? It can be rationalized, perhaps treated as a humorous incident. Or, since the problem in his own eye is invisible, the person may blame others for the communication block. The resultant attitude that "nobody can understand me and nobody is speaking intelligibly," can attain paranoid proportions. Perhaps these bizarre events are brought on because the critical area for semantic-syntactic operations lies close to the "feeling brain." The damage responsible for the language disorder may also encroach upon this structure to produce the perplexing emotional indifference to the severe illness.

The severest derangement of the semantic-syntactic mechanism is one which produces "jargon aphasia," an intermittent or continuously unintelligible babble. Although speech is spontaneous, fluent, and replete with emotionally expressive intonation, the sound sequences become so scrambled that they make no sense. Yet, unlike an infant's babbling, the sounds are only those of the patient's native language. An occasional sequence may be repeated so often that it seems like a newly invented word, hence the term "neologistic jargon." The damage to the mechanism is so complete that it ceases to exert control over the output program. When an urge to speak releases the articulation mechanism it "runs free," exhibiting its intrinsic, ingrained habits—meaningless but highly structured sound sequences. The above explanation is speculative. It has recently been observed that jargon patients tend to be older than other aphasics. Advanced age increases the possibility of multiple damage sites due to "mini-strokes." Therefore, the cause of the jargon may be more complex.

7

Clay's Communication Disorder

Clay's case history possesses many of the features just described in the last chapter yet is unlike any one of them. This suggests minor damage to several components of the language mechanism rather than major damage to any single one.

On admission to the hospital he was at his worst, as are most patients immediately following a stroke. The brain, like any injured organ, overreacts. It recoils in the face of assault and throws up all its defenses. Since emergency reponses of the body are rather exaggerated, they often make the patient look much sicker than he really is. Take a commonplace example. A mosquito bite on one side of the face near the eye can swell the face to lopsided proportions. This tends to close the eye and thus protect it. But why such an outpouring of fluid beneath the skin, as if to begrudge the poor insect the involuntary donation of a few drops of blood? The skin reaction seems excessive only from the myopic vantage point of a single bite.

The wisdom of the body incorporates the survival mechanisms of the species. It is always prepared for mayhem. Look at a mosquito bite from the skin's point of view. How is the skin to know that this particular onslaught will only be a single bite and not a thousand bites from a cloud of mosquitoes? The memory of human evolution, which is built into body chemistry, necessarily dictates a conservative strategy. Longterm goals such as survival of the species subordinate cosmetics to longevity, and vision takes priority over facial symmetry. The eye must be protected at all cost.

The same state of affairs occurs with an acute brain injury. The brain goes into shock, and is temporarily "out of order." As if likely in Clay's case, a shower of tiny plaques was released from a large artery in the left side of his neck, and became lodged in the progressively narrower brain arteries downstream. Only a small amount of brain tissue was actually deprived of blood supply by this accident, but the surrounding healthy tissue reacted like the skin surrounding a mosquito bite—with massive swelling and a spasm of unblocked neighboring arteries. The result was a temporary shutdown of brain function which extended far beyond the actual area of damage. Recall that the brain is encased in a rigid, bony skull and can't swell too much without putting pressure on itself—which could compound the original problem. This is the reason that Clay was given cortisone injections in the hospital. This hormone affects the emergency reactions of the body in such a way as to reduce swelling.

Where was the initial injury? It is identified in the very beginning of his story in Chapter One. He first gagged on food, then the right side of his face and his right arm became weak and he couldn't speak. There was a brief recovery period, but the stroke progressed during the night. However, he remained conscious and capable of understanding other people's speech to some extent. He was sufficiently in touch with the world and his situation to get to bed, to make a probable diagnosis, and to check his face in the mirror. This cluster of symptoms marks the location of the primary damage—it involved the *output* channels for arm, face, mouth, and throat movements in the left side of the brain. Immediately adjacent to these areas are the output programs that convert verbally conceived images into spoken or written messages. We've described how all these areas are in the front part of the left side of the brain.

Fortunately, all the *input* areas are in the rear, as are the syntactic-semantic mechanisms. That is why he could understand and conceive of a reply but not produce it. The only verbal message he was able to get out was the somewhat primitive written utterance, "weedee, weedee." This was, of course, a highly condensed, personal, and poignant message to Jane, who shared the world knowledge necessary to understand it. However, the remainder of his messages had to be in the form of pantomime. Thus, he could answer the question "Who is Jane?" by pointing to her and then making an embracing gesture of his arms which meant, "She is my wife." When the nurse asked, "Are you right-handed?" he couldn't answer verbally, but could nod and hold up his right arm in answer. He naturally switched his mode of communication to nonverbal output channels. He sensed these to be intact. They were the route through which his residual comprehension of incoming messages, his internal needs, and his unimpaired knowledge of the world could be communicated to others. He could cope.

But a series of surprises was in store for him. Recall that he could distinguish between his right and left hands but couldn't imagine which foot was which. This is reminiscent of a child who learns that "the right hand is the one you eat with," an idea which may antedate the more general concept of a right and left side of the body. He was puzzled by the temporary loss of this abstract concept. In the American Revolution, illiterate, rural army recruits were taught to march by tieing hay to their left foot and straw to their right. The drill sergeant would then chant the cadence "hay–foot, straw–foot" instead of "left, right." He and Jane were about to rediscover what every one-year-old infant knows; namely, that highly symbolic communication can be carried out by means of visual and auditory inputs and gestural outputs, that bypass the speech mechanisms in the left side of the brain. Recall that Clay could watch his uninterested nurse like a hawk the first night in the hospital and understand her attitude. The next day he could watch a basketball game on TV and follow the plays. These activities drew heavily on the special skills of his undamaged right side of the brain

—facial-emotional recognition and spatial perception. But the moment he tried to read a newspaper, he discovered that he could see but not comprehend the headlines. This visual input called upon certain highly specialized mechanisms in the left side of the brain. Unlike the visual images of hospital personnel or basketball players, the headlines in the newspaper were not *pictures of real events*. Rather, they were a *visual code for speech patterns*. This was the first clear evidence of brain damage that extended backward from the primarily involved output mechanisms. We don't know whether there was a small clot that had also lodged in the rear of the left side of his brain, or whether it was the spasm and swelling that had spread. In any event, reading was impaired along with speech output, and the stage was set for the next fiasco.

Jane is a professional educator, so she naturally thought, "My husband cannot speak, but can comprehend *my speech*. He can communicate nonverbally by charades and by pointing to objects. He's just verbally 'locked in' as it were. I'll show him a chart of the alphabet and he'll spell out his verbal messages." The very first experiment showed that spelling, performed by pointing to printed letters, was an impaired as speaking and reading ability. All three tasks involve the verbal machinery in addition to nonverbal gestures and world knowledge. Clay saw the alphabet clearly and pointed with confidence. Was his visual analyzer disconnected from an intact semantic-syntactic mechanism? We might conclude this if auditory comprehension of spoken language was normal. However, it wasn't.

Evidence for this included his inability to carry out complex verbal commands such as, "Place your right index finger on your left ear," although he could accurately carry out simpler commands such as, "Raise your right hand." He also tells us that certain complex sentences were hard to comprehend, those containing double negatives for example. Furthermore, he was delighted by the TV presentation of Sesame Street during the first few months of recovery. The creators of this educational program have gone to great lengths to present verbal information in highly simplified form for children. The verbal messages are reinforced by animation, which made maximum use of the undamaged right side of his brain. His preference for the program suggests a limited ability to handle complex verbal inputs that taxed the semantic-syntactic mechanisms. During recovery, evidence of this problem accumulated.

Five months after the stroke he telephoned to discuss this manuscript. He still complained that prolonged phone conversations were physically tiring. The surprise in the conversation was his deliberate statement: "I have finished . . . or by the end of the week I will have finished, getting my notes together." This was startling because it was typical of his sentences prior to the stroke. It illustrated a complexity of sentence structure that had been noticeably absent since the illness began. His speaking style had paralleled his preference for simplified listening materials.

One of the most telling signs of a comprehension deficiency was his inability to notice his obvious aphasic speech errors. On reciting the alphabet, while counting on his knuckles, he would repeatedly say "Q, U, R, S, T, U, V," and continue merrily to the end, only to be surprised that there were twenty-seven letters instead of twenty-six. The letter "Q" never appears in English unless followed by the letter "U." This was such an ingrained habit that he could not say the letter "Q" without saying "U" right after it. He would then continue the equally automatic habit of the alphabet sequence with "R, S, T, U, V," etc. In a literate adult, these habits are programmed. In Clay's case, this program was occasionally running free, somewhat disconnected from his linguistic intentions. He would also point out directions to Jane who was driving the car, but say "Turn left" while pointing appropriately to the right. He was sending contradictory messages, one from each half of the brain. Reading maps and pointing out directions drew upon the spatial skills of his intact right brain and he was accurate. But simultaneous verbal expression invoked the semantic skills of the left brain which unfortunately produced not the target word, but a word which was closely associated with the one intended. The point we are making is that he didn't *register* the error, and was equally amazed by the resultant confusion.

Still another example of impaired self-monitoring occurred while he was casually describing routine family preparations for minor illnesses. In context, the intended sentence was, "You've lived long enough that you keep a thermometer in the house." But the words "in your mouth" replaced the words "in the house." Usually, Clay relishes verbal puns. The substitution of "mouth" for "house" had at least three motivations: it expressed his fear of being chronically, and aphasically, ill; it was indeed another place you could keep a thermometer; and it rhymed with the intended word. Knowing how sensitive psychoanalysts are to "Freudian slips," it is particularly significant that he neither noticed the substitution nor appreciated the pun. It is also of interest that Sigmund Freud wrote a book on aphasia prior to his invention of psychoanalysis.

Even after fluent speech had returned, the defective linkage between the semantic-syntactic mechanism and the output programs persisted. These two components must coordinate in the generation of speech and writing. Seven months after the stroke, when Clay clearly knew the sentences to be expressed, the intended words "store window" came out as "straw window," and "witchcraft" came out as "witchcrap." In discussing a mutual friend who had had open heart surgery and a kidney infection, the word "infection" came out as "inspection." As we've explained, many of these sound substitutions make sense, just as the unintentional whole word substitutions do. The errors are not random. The words "right" and "left" are strongly associated in the mind. Clay did have a derogatory opinion of witchcraft. The heart of the friend with the kidney infection was indeed being inspected. But he made these errors much more frequently than would be expected from normal "slips of the tongue." And he was often unaware of these errors when conversation was animated.

When speaking carefully however, he might notice an error and correct himself, leading him to predict recurrent difficulties and devise strategies for circumventing them. For example, "disability policy" was a real tongue twister and was replaced by "disability insurance." "Extremely" was replaced by "very." In pronouncing the medical term "vertebral," Clay accented the first syllable (ver′ tĕ bral) instead of accenting the second syllable (ver tē′ bral) as he had done before the stroke. It is well-known that damage to the output program causes particular problems with unaccented initial syllables (ex treme′ ly, ver tē′ bral), but much less difficulty with accented initial syllables (ve′ ry, ver′ te bral). Clay discovered this phenomenon spontaneously. And rather than say "enter tain′ guests," he preferred "give′ a par′ty."

A much more serious defect of the semantic-syntactic mechanism itself was his persistent problem in naming. Nouns are low frequency words in the vocabulary. All of us have an occasional word on "the tip of the tongue" which we instantly recognize when supplied by somebody else. But this rarely happens at the dinner table with words such as knife, fork, spoon, salt, or pepper. One strategy used to circumvent this problem was to substitute the general word "thing" for the missing noun and to simultaneously point to the object. This preserved fluency, but was obviously an impossible strategy in a telephone conversation, or when the object wasn't physically present. Another was to talk around the name; for example, "I need one of those small curved things you use to stir sugar in coffee." Clay used both strategies. The first led Jane to comment that he used the word "thing" too often. The second is illustrated by these excerpts from his dictated notes:

When three people are in the room with me and two of them are carrying on a conversation, I am unable to clear their conversation out and so it ruins the conversation with the person I am talking with. This has always been a problem such as at cocktail parties. I'm usually not able to clear the person I am not listening to out.

After reading a sentence containing a double negative he dictated:

That was a very hard sentence. I think what made it hard was the "not" that switched things around. I've noticed that before, in reading. That they switch things around by putting "not" in there and it's difficult for me to—well, let's put it this way: it's much more difficult than a simple . . . statement of fact. The reason I paused is that I was trying to think of . . . the word "imperative." (He means "declarative.")

Note the relative informational poverty of the sentences and the profusion of small function words; the very opposite of telegrammatic speech which is concise and pithy. We've described this pattern previously in more exaggerated form—in the case of a patient suffering from severe syntactic-semantic damage. It was mild in Clay's case and only surfaced after he had regained normal speech fluency. Recovery of the output mechanisms was very rapid, and the above passage was dictated only a month after the stroke.

A quantitative study of these dictated notes was undertaken in an attempt to document some of the subtleties of the recovery process. We compared twelve hundred words dictated a month after the stroke with an equal number of words dictated nine months later. It was of some interest that the most frequent word used early in recovery was the pronoun "I," reflecting Clay's admitted self-preoccupation at that time. In the later sample, this word had receded to third place, and was outstripped in frequency by the words "in" and "the." His interests were turning outward. We were surprised to find that the number of different words in the vocabulary had increased only slightly—about four percent. But the average length of the words had definitely increased over the nine-month recovery period. For example, one month after the stroke only two five-syllable words were used (incidentally and considerably). Nine months later, the speech sample showed ten words of this length (psychotherapy, inevitably, psychotherapist, international, psychotherapist's, occasionally, documentary, possibility, constitutional, neurological), one word of six syllables (hospitalization), and one of seven syllables (inevitability). Concurrently, the percentage of monosyllabic words dropped by seven percent, so there was an overall shift of vocabulary balance toward the longer words. As noted earlier, his sentence structure was also becoming more complex throughout this period.

Although subtle, and occurring over the course of many months, these very gradual changes are typical of the recovery process in aphasia. Here are transcripts from another patient—describing the same photograph at two points in time during convalescence. One month after the stroke: sixteen percent polysyllabic words (in italics).

Well, all I know is *somebody* is *clipping* the *kreples* and same why, *someone* here on the *kureping* arm . . . why, I don't know. And then you got, a this flot to tell them right see. Now this here I'm *confoy* here *because* the have *explained* what I don't know.

Fifteen months after the stroke: twenty-seven percent polysyllabic words (in italics).

There is a man *plowing* a field and on one side of the, oh, field is his *apparently* wife *leaning* up *against* the tree. And there is a *very attractive* girl. I'd *assume* they're his *daughter*. He is not *exactly* a *very* fine *looking* house. There's no *other evidence* to use a *story* at this *moment*.

The similarities to our findings in Clay's case are striking. Small increases in the proportion of polysyllabic words are liable to go unnoticed during the heartbreakingly slow recovery period, submerged as they are in hundreds of words, each a precious message from a mind seeking to relocate itself. Special attention to such increments, commonly paid when a baby first begins to talk, should add to the hope and optimism of the aphasic's family.

It is tempting to attribute these changes to the slow recovery of the semantic-syntactic mechanism. After all, fluency was essentially recovered, albeit via dodges and strategies, by the time our first speech sample was dictated a month after the stroke. However, the brain works as a whole. The language mechanism does not respect the neat diagrams of its components that we draw for purposes of exposition. Even isolated damage to an output component changes our relationship to the environment—the input patterns selected and the output patterns attempted.

Any loss of function gives us a whole new set of problems. Imagine that you are a skier who develops a weak leg. Reports of snow and ski conditions, which previously captured your attention, have a profoundly different meaning now that a ski trip is out of the question. The reports may become even more salient if you decide to ski vicariously in the imagination. Or, they may become irrelevant and uninteresting if your plans turn to other pursuits. In either case, the world looks different. The height of a curb or a threshold becomes a problem to be negotiated consciously; a problem which was barely noticed previously and was solved unconsciously. In the same way, Clay's output limitations certainly constricted the complexity of the things he tried to say, and perhaps even the things he thought.

Commonly, in cases of aphasia, the output mechanisms for writing recover more slowly than those for speaking. That is why Clay had to dictate this manuscript. At first, he had trouble even copying a written pattern, but the ability to write began to return in the hospital. At that time, he wrote the name of his best friend and misspelled it. He knew it looked wrong but did not know why. Even a year and a half following the stroke a scribbled note shows letter reversals in two words: "hypertensive" is spelled "hypersentive," and "normal" is spelled "mornal." The errors were not corrected as they usually are, so they were presumably not noticed. Thus, most of the errors that have disappeared from speech still crop up in writing. This clearly implicates the output program for writing because the semantic-syntactic mechanisms function properly for speech.

Clay's numerical problems were also part of his aphasia. Numbers suffuse our daily living in myriad guises. Counting things, writing checks, paying carfare, reading recipes, shopping, pushing buttons in elevators, knowing the date, year, and time of day, knowing street addresses, telephone numbers, and people's ages; these are but a few of the most common.

Thinking in numbers is a different process than thinking in sentences. Children learn to count on their fingers and some people never outgrow this—they still use finger movements as a memory device, a portable calculator when doing arithmetic. Others give this up and rely on visual images—for example, a staircase consisting of nine steps with the tenth being a landing, and another nine steps with the twentieth being the second landing, etc. Subtracting three from twenty-two means descending two steps to the second landing, then descending one more step to the nineteenth step. Other people don't use either of these strategies but handle the internal calculation quite abstractly. Thus, there are wide differences in the way people do mental arithmetic. In general, the outside world only cares about the final answer, and not the method by which it was achieved; in computation, the end justifies the means. In verbal thought however, society is more interested in the way conclusions are arrived at. Even the desired answer may not be trusted. Aphasic difficulty with numbers is therefore more poorly understood than corresponding difficulty with words and sentences. The problem begins to make sense when broken down into component skills such as:

a) Problems with the *concept of number itself*, an abstract skill which is part of what we have called world knowledge.

b) Problems in *naming numbers;* that is, problems in assigning verbal labels to abstract number concepts. (For example, the words "one, two, three" or "first, second, third.")

c) Problems in writing numbers as a memory aid—for most people a requirement in long division.

d) Problems in *spatially* manipulating numbers, either in the mind (visual imagery) or on paper—for example linging up the digits for the following problem for example.

```
  234              234
-  14   versus   -14
 ----             ----
  220               94
```

e) Problems in simply remembering what stage you are at and what to do next while solving some arithmetic problem.

Clay's self-imposed exercises to help recover speech included the virtually automatic skill of counting, and we've seen the initial difficulty he had in formulating the word "ten." The fact that he overcame the block by verbalizing a synonym (the digits "one-oh") proves that the basic number concept was intact, and that name assignment was the problem. In the same way, he worked out a strategy for roughly converting prices in Danish kroner (about twenty cents) to dollars—dividing by five. He also worked out the equivalent strategy of dropping the last digit (dividing by ten) and then multiplying by two $\left(\frac{2}{10}=\frac{1}{5}\right)$ But he had difficulty implementing either strategy, presumably a simpler task, since he could neither divide by five nor multiply by two. Certainly, basic arithmetic concepts were intact. What then was the problem? We did a small experiment.

Joe: "I'll write a multiplication problem on paper, and you do it in your head."

$$\begin{array}{r} 74 \\ \times\ 2 \\ \hline \end{array}$$

Clay: "First, it's 7 times 4. Then, you have to remember the 8. Next, it's 7 times 2, which is 14. The answer is 148."

He was obviously carrying out the correct operations and indeed got the right answer. But the words he uttered concurrently didn't correspond to his mental operations. While multiplying 2 by 4 he said "7 times 4," but nevertheless he got the correct answer, 8. Nor did he realize the discrepancy.

That was nine months after the stroke. For the first three months he couldn't even copy numbers correctly, nor could he write them correctly from dictation, although he was able to repeat (echo) spoken digits verbally and read them aloud. This accounts for the difficulty he had in writing checks, and with arithmetic problems that could not be done mentally (for example, long division, which requires written output as a memory aid).

Finally, part of his arithmetic problem was due to a sheer memory and concentration difficulty. Thus, in attempting the problem of starting at 100 and serially subtracting 7's "in his head" (100, 93, 86, 79, etc.) he was flustered and demoralized. This happens to be a standard bedside test used by every hospital neuropsychiatrist, and one that he had administered many times. Most people take a bit more time getting from 93 to 86 and from 86 to 79 than they do getting from 100 to 93 or from 79 to 72. Why is this? Crossing a boundary of ten involves three steps for many people:

$$\text{Problem: } 93 - 7 = ?$$
$$\text{Step 1) } 7 = 3 + 4$$
$$\text{Step 2) } 93 - 3 = 90$$
$$\text{Step 3) } 90 - 4 = 86$$

In contrast, 79 minus 7 is intuitively seen to lie between the boundaries of 80 and 70. Thus, it reduces to the simpler problem of $9 - 7$, and the answer 72 is usually reached in one step. The rhythm of the successive spoken answers betrays this strategy, since a three-step calculation takes longer than a one-step calculation.

This problem was exaggerated in Clay's case and further compounded by two other difficulties. He would often say a number which was different from the one he had just calculated. Unfortunately, he sometimes heard himself say it, and then used the erroneous answer as the starting point for the next subtraction. The result was disastrous. It seems ridiculous to point out that each new subtraction of a 7 begins with the last answer and wipes the mental slate clean of the previous calculation. But Clay reported a peculiar difficulty in this necessary shift of attention which we take so much for granted. His surprising description of his mental operations on this test follows:

Joe: How do you actually do it?
Clay: Start with 100. Then, 100 minus 7 is 93.
Joe: How?
Clay: Instantly, it just is!

Joe: Okay, continue.
Clay: Next is 93 minus 7. *But first you have to forget 100.*

This insightful comment qualifies what we usually mean by
memory problems in an important way. He seemed to be
having difficulty forgetting parts of the task that were no
longer relevant.

In summary, Clay had no difficulties with number concepts or with their spatial manipulation (the latter is probably
a right brain function). However, there was a defect in writing the number correctly and in naming it verbally. It would
seem that numerical errors could be triggered by having
named them incorrectly—that the erroneous word intruded
upon the calculation process. Also, there were general problems of memory and attention-shifting in complex calculations. The net effort was a persistent problem with arithmetic
skills which outlasted the speech difficulty. This showed up
in many disturbing ways that frequently involved money.

Money is a universal language, and current events more
often than not involve currency. That the computational
hang-up played havoc with financial aspects of Clay's public
and private life has been amply documented. But perhaps
more intriguing than the horrors of the disability are the
ingenious strategies which can be invented for coping. Some
are so simple that they hardly bear mention. If you can't
check a grocery bill or compute the sales tax on a purchase,
you can trust the salesperson. People aren't usually out to get
you, and cheating by overcharging sales tax on small pur-
chases is a tough way to make a living. Another way is to
carry an electronic pocket calculator, one of the most inex-
pensive brain prostheses. You can ask the salesperson to write
out your personal check, and then proofread it before you
sign it. Or, ask the waiter to add a fifteen percent tip to the
check and kindly add it up. The possibilities are endless, but
most of them involve a recasting of one's attitude towards
others in financial transactions. This necessitates a change in
one's self-concept.

The final group of aphasic symptoms deals with a damaged

brain's lowered efficiency in processing information. We all have limits, and when life becomes too complicated we experience a sensation of drowning or being swamped. This is technically known as "information overload." Many of Clay's social disasters in the recovery period had to do with this phenomenon. His brain was easily overloaded by complex verbal information, and when the limit was exceeded he felt panicky, confused, and fatigued. This was compounded by the embarrassing fact that information overload occurred in many situations in which he had formerly been competent. Among them were the intricate plots of detective stories, the maze of traffic signs at busy superhighway intersections, filling out forms for a passport, instructions for replacing the head of an electric razor, and so on. As speech began to recover, he sent people on multiple errands to the same place—much to their annoyance—since he could only ask for (think of?) one thing at a time.

One of the most interesting symptoms of reduced information processing efficiency was conversational. After the stroke, Clay found it very difficult to tune out an irrelevant voice and focus his complete attention upon a single verbal message. Thus, he became intolerant of noisy parties where voices had to be sorted out. He fatigued quickly and withdrew.

Another aspect of this new intolerance for competing verbal messages was his incredible sensitivity to interruption, much more than simple irritation over a breach of etiquette. Most of us are mildly offended when interrupted by our listener. Our speech may falter momentarily, but our minds don't go blank. Yet this was one of Clay's problems early in the recovery process. Conversational interruptions while he was speaking might precipitate a memory wipeout—he would forget what he was trying to say. This phenomenon is an exaggeration of normal functioning. It constitutes the best evidence that the semantic-syntactic mechanism in the brain for both producing and understanding sentences is one and the same. When this mechanism is tuned to the input analyzers and thus to the other person's intentions, we can understand speech but momentarily cannot speak. This configuration is commonly known as the "listening state." When it is tuned to our own intentions and to our output programs we can speak, but we cannot simultaneously understand others. This configuration is the "speaking state." The brain cannot function in both states at once.

Clay's sensitivity to interruption is an exaggeration of this universal feature of conversation. While he was speaking, his linguistic machinery was working with great effort—at top efficiency. Lacking reserves, it was particularly vulnerable. An interruption by his listener (a competing verbal message) preempted the semantic-syntactic mechanism, throwing it into the listening state. In this new configuration it was disconnected from his original intention and from the output mechanisms. He not only stopped speaking, but he could not resume speaking on the same topic when the interruption was over.

Perhaps the mild difficulty he experienced when reading aloud related to this phenomenon; comprehension seemed better during silent reading. It is possible that even his own voice interfered with concurrent linguistic analysis.

Thus, we see that aphasia lays bare the organization of the normal brain and teaches us a great deal about the peculiar way in which we have evolved as verbally conversing creatures.

8

The Aphasic
as Psychiatrist

Aphasia is perhaps the most disabling illness for a psychiatrist. It would have been possible to continue my practice with loss of limbs, eyesight, or other functions, but not with loss of speech and memory. Psychiatric treatment basically involves language and communication.

One psychotherapist I know has a severe one-sided facial paralysis—worse than mine—and does very good work. Another resourceful therapist suddenly became deaf following a virus disease, but retained his power of speech. He had to decide if he could continue his work, so he suggested that his patients might try the experiement of writing their communication in his office. Some wanted to try, and said it worked out quite well. Less time was spent on irrelevant chitchat because handwriting was slower than speech. He could also observe certain emotions in their faces which might have been different had they been talking, such as biting a cheek, sweating over words they were writing, hesitation in their writing, erasures, slips of the pen, and hand tremors. Since he was able to comment when necessary, he felt it was a good, though not ideal, way of functioning as a psychotherapist.

My work consists of listening, watching, remembering, sorting the significant from the insignificant in my patients' comments, asking questions, and occasionally making a pertinent comment. I must recognize my patient's emotions and respond, at least internally, to these emotions as well as his words. This has been described as participant observation. I listen as my patient describes his anxieties, depressions, phobias, and the various experiences he has in living. I must try to feel a little of what he feels (participation). The patient is the focus of my attention. I must be sufficiently involved with the patient's life to be able to think about him, to mentally replay our sessions together, to discover recurring themes, and to see his problems within a larger framework of psychoanalytic thought.

I must also remember what the patient told me in order to connect it to what follows, even though what follows may not be in logical sequence. If the sequence were logical, I would have no function; the patient could connect it himself. Memory is essential for the analyst who tries to fit the pieces of the puzzle together, seeking to discover patterns of behavior, recurring anxieties which patients have in their relations with others, and the kinds of experiences which cause problems in living.

My own training as a psychoanalyst required that I be analyzed. I learned what it is like, and as a result I am in a better position to empathize with a patient. Webster defines empathy in terms similar to sympathy, but psychotherapists tend to use the word in a somewhat different fashion. Hinsie and Campbell's *Psychiatric Dictionary* define it as "putting oneself into the psychological frame of reference of another, so that the other person's thinking, feeling, and acting are understood and to some extent, predictable." Perhaps sympathy is "feeling for" someone else, while empathy is "feeling with" the other person.

An example of empathy occurred during transcription of the tapes I dictated for this book. In my early tapes I was struggling painfully with speech. They were ghastly to listen to. My friend Mercedes had offered to transcribe them, but kept making excuses for her delay along with promises to do them soon. I suspect that she couldn't do them because she was too personally involved with me, and emotionally affected by the tapes. That would be empathy—feeling with me.

Another typist whom I had never met also worked on the tapes. She reported that listening to me and to Jane on some tapes was quite trying; at times she found it very hard to continue. She was probably empathizing.

To empathize it is necessary to have an experience more or less like that of the other person. Most of us have felt pain, frustration, and rejection, and may be able to empathize with these feelings. We can also sympathize, or even deny the feelings.

Obviously, one cannot have the identical experience of another person. But once we have matured enough to see that others are as human as we are, we can empathize with feelings which are common to a variety of experiences—pain, humiliation, shame, joy, or happiness. For instance, as a man I cannot experience being a woman, but I can psychoanalyze a woman and empathize with her rage, shame or whatever. I don't know what a woman feels during orgasm, but I probably know more about it than a woman who has never had an orgasm. I can never know childbirth but I know pain and joy, and I can learn something about it by listening to women's descriptions.

The best illustration of empathy is the following description of an animal experiment. Two young monkeys were in separate soundproof rooms with a soundproof glass between them. They could see but not hear each other. Laboratory monkeys are easily trained to press a bar to get food. The first monkey (Abraham) presses a bar—food appears for Abraham, and the second monkey (Isaac) receives an electric shock. Abraham eats; Isaac jumps around and makes strange faces (remember—no sound).

If we anthropomorphize a bit, we can say that Abraham

thinks there's a crazy monkey on the other side of the glass and continues to press the bar and eat while Isaac makes crazy gestures.

Abraham, *who has never been shocked*, and Isaac are now shifted in position, and Isaac has the food bar. Abraham is in the hot seat. Isaac presses the bar, gets food, and Abraham jumps and acts crazy. After this happens a few times, Isaac remembers the shock. He knows that when he presses the bar, something terrible happens to Abraham—he empathizes and therefore can predict what Abraham will feel and do. The surprising thing is that Isaac stops pressing the bar and therefore stops eating. He cannot eat and commit this sin. If the experiment is repeated with Abraham and another naive monkey, Abraham will also starve himself.

Fortunately the experiment has never been carried on long enought to reach the point of extreme starvation. Experimenters have empathy too. It does show that an experience of some similar sort is necessary to share another's experience. This does not mean that all humans are like monkeys and will respond sensitively; maybe not even all monkeys do. And one need not have had electric shock to share the experience of pain and terror; having felt these emotions at some time we can empathize with them in another.

Empathy is the stock in trade of my kind of psychotherapy. If I can feel what another person feels, I may be able to predict what the other person may do and feel, and may, in some sense, help him or make him feel that he's not all alone.

The psychotherapist's awareness of another person's feelings must be communicated with no sense of condemnation to his fragile self-esteem. This enables further communication to follow, allowing him to tell you more about his life, and this will occur without the exhausting problems of power struggles or fruitless efforts at persuasion.

There is a tendency to think that communication (in psychotherapy and elsewhere) is mainly verbal. Although it may not be true that actions always speak louder than words, many subtle actions have a profound and frequently unknowable effect. In psychotherapy, obvious motions such as a smile, a raised eyebrow, or a restless movement may communicate—sometimes unintentionally. For this reason, it is incumbent upon the therapist to try to make his communications explicit. I say "try" because it is often impossible.

I have been haunted for years by an example of a failure in explicit communication. I had a patient who had come to the United States from Poland about twenty years earlier. During one of her narratives I remarked, "That was a funny thing to say," meaning peculiar or strange. Six months later I learned she was greatly hurt because she thought that by "funny" I meant "laughable." These are frequent occurrences and the doctor is often not told about them. It's one reason why therapists tend toward silence—but even that is a form communication (as is a poker face) and may be interpreted as boredom.

While I am listening to the patient I must also listen to my own thoughts, and I must then decide whether these thoughts would be valid to communicate to my patient, or whether it would be better to omit them. Will they facilitate or interfere with our communication?

Let me give an example. A patient tells me about a sudden anger he feels with his wife or friend. I ask him what preceded this and he says, "Nothing." I pursue it, and say "Something must have happened." He then tells me about a seemingly minor incident. Suddenly in my own mind I have a fantasy of my first wife and an incident leading to my divorce. I know this means that he has triggered a memory that is *somewhat* similar in emotional content to his encounter with his wife or friend. I don't tell him what my memory was, but I do make the connection between the incident he related and his anger. If I'm lucky he may tell me that I "hit the nail on the thumb."

Patients' reactions to me derive from their observations of me or their own past history and fantasies. Often their view of me is not consistent with reality; a young woman once asked me if I had suddenly turned grey because she always perceived me as a blond—clearly, her desire to see me as a younger man. Other patients see the doctor as some sort of godlike figure—a magical helper.

Some patients resist both therapy and the doctor, holding back things which will make them feel uncomfortable—anxieties which are causing the problems. Since much of psychotherapy is communication, patients often have to learn how to talk freely. In all other relationships they have learned that there are usually certain taboo subjects—"not nice," "poor taste," inappropriate, or offensive. In the therapeutic relationship the patient has to know that there are no holds barred; he *should* in fact say whatever he is thinking about. With a reticent patient, I may ask some provocative questions, such as "Why don't you look at me when you arrive or leave; are you afraid I'll see something?" or "Why do you wear so much perfume; are you being enticing or do you think you smell or I smell?" Unless the patient learns to be free and open, we cannot reach the anxieties which are problematic.

This may evoke new emotions in the relationship—anger, hate, resentment, whatever. It usually does not mean, however, that we end up disliking each other.

I do not form immediate likes or dislikes to many people. Within a few days however, I do have some sort of positive or negative emotional reaction to a patient. It is possible to do psychotherapeutic work with someone whom one dislikes, but, if one is going to spend a good deal of time with a person, it is easier to have friendly feelings toward him. It's also easier if the patient has some sort of friendly feelings toward his therapist although, of course, he's free to feel whatever he wishes. A patient, for instance, who is never angry at anyone has a serous problem; it is something we work on in his therapy—what aborts the anger?

Dependency upon the therapist is to some degree encouraged, but the long-term effort is to foster individual autonomy. Interruptions of treatment can be useful in helping patients understand their ability to get along on their own. This is usually the result of routine vacations, out-of-town professional meetings, and the like. In my case it came as a result of illness.

There is a general belief that "Doctors shouldn't get sick." This is particularly true if the patient feels that the doctor is some sort of god. Unfortunately, doctors are mortal, and every one of my patients found this out.

When I first went into the hospital, Jane checked my appointment book and telephoned my patients. She told them that I would have to cancel for a short time because I was ill.

Jane: We knew very little in the first few days about Clay's prognosis and I didn't know how much to tell the patients. I said he was ill and in the hospital for some tests. It left them all very unsatisfied, but I promised to call them back within a few days, which I did. Then I could be more specific with each one of them.

My patients had many responses to my illness and, as will be seen from their reports, highly individual responses to me. I suspect that it would be hard to get a consistent picture of me from their accounts. One patient was, at the time, extremely upset for reasons other than my illness. She told Jane that she was referred to me by someone else, and since I had only seen her for about two months she went back to the other therapist. None of my other patients were feeling this kind of emergency, although there were various special problems. Fortunately one patient was out of town for a few days and another had cancelled the next appointment, so Jane could speak to them after I began to recover.

What follows are accounts by some of my patients of the problems of having a psychiatrist who had suffered an acute illness and was aphasic.

Fred

Fred was a fifty-three-year-old man suffering from a severe depression following his company's move from New York to California. He was forced to move with them, and that's when the depression started. When he saw me he was border-

ing on suicide and we worked together for about nine
months. He was improving rapidly and was starting to make
trips to California in preparation for his final move. The impending move again brought up, in minor forms, the old
depressive symptoms. I had just returned from the hospital
and didn't know what I could do. He had confidence in me;
he couldn't fill another doctor in in such a short time, and
develop confidence in him. He was going to leave in another
month. So, I told him in my halting speech that I didn't
know what I could do for him but would see him a few times
on an as-needed basis. I think I saw him three times, and saw
his wife perhaps once during this period.

Since I couldn't convince myself that I was able to be of
any value to anybody, I couldn't in conscience charge him,
but I asked him and his wife to write their reactions to the situation. An edited version follows:

The first is from his wife, Harriet, whom I had seen several times. Both reactions were written just before leaving the
East—eight weeks poststroke.

When Mrs. Dahlberg called to cancel Fred's appointment because
of tests Dr. Dahlberg was undergoing at the hospital, my first reaction was one of thankfulness that Fred was scheduled to be away for
a while and therefore would not feel that he was "missing" appointments.

Before Dr. Dahlberg called, I kept wondering what was wrong
and I thought of our regard for him. I was concerned for Dr. Dahlberg and for Fred—and how he would react if his doctor was really
ill.

When Mrs. Dahlberg called and informed me of his condition, my
reaction was shock and foreboding. I knew that there were only two
people Fred could freely talk to—his psychiatrist and me. I wondered if I could carry more of the "burden."

I tried to minimize the shock by emphasizing a "minor" stroke.
However, the next few days were very, very bad. The California
trip had not gone well—Fred was upset and frightened. When we
saw Dr. Dahlberg, I did fear that Fred was beginning to slide into
another breakdown. After the session, Fred's condition was much
calmer because of his utter trust and confidence in his doctor. The

fact that his doctor had some speech impairment did not make any difference.

Now, he holds on to the thought that he can contact his doctor by mail or telephone—if he must. Whether Fred consults a psychiatrist in California or not, I know that he will always consider Dr. Dahlberg "his doctor."

From Fred:

Before I discuss my reaction to Dr. Dahlberg's stroke, I would like to provide some background.

I was panicked about getting a new job in California. My wife and I made two trips in the spring to California with favorable results. We shortly decided that we would rejoin the company out west. Dr. Dahlberg said I should no longer consider myself "sick" in regard to the original breakdown. We had entered into new phases of analysis which both he and I recognized as being important to my well-being and happiness, namely my family relationships, especially with my daughters.

Thursday evening, just after my last trip to California, I was notified by phone that Dr. Dahlberg could not see me for my regularly scheduled appointment on Friday since he was in the hospital, having suffered a mild stroke. This news came just prior to my plans for taking another trip by myself, for the first time without Harriet.

My initial reaction was worry about its effect on him, not on me. I was saddened and grieved that it happened to an individual whom I held in high esteem, and with whom over the past seven to eight months I had developed both a bond of kinship and deep friendship. Really, I felt that there are only two people who understand me— Harriet and Dr. Dahlberg.

It was only after I became ill that I understood the ills and needs of others who were ill, and the fact that there were people like Dr. Dahlberg who had a lot to give and did give to make people well.

It had not really dawned on me that I had lost my psychiatrist, my relief valve, my advisor, and my friend because I thought I was "quite well" and would soon be off to California.

Still, the trip I had just returned from was very wearing on me and I felt panicky and almost on the verge of not being able to cope. I was glad to get home to my family.

Saturday and Sunday I was a bundle of nerves and close to panic. These last days made me think about the loss of my psychiatrist and my need to discuss my feelings with him. Even though I knew he had been ill, I talked to Harriet and found out that he was out of the hospital. Although not practicing, maybe I could see him. I knew I wanted to see him and had to see him. I called and got an appointment. I believe it was at this time that he advised I take some valium and relax for a couple of days. I totally recognized my need to discuss my feelings with him, and was trying to push and impose to get more of his time.

Over the past weeks I have managed to see him once a week, but really would have wanted it to be more. During this period, when I'm no longer "quite well" and the deadline for the move approaches, I am desperately aware that I have lost the time of my doctor and friend who could have advised me and reassured me that this move and the future, although uncertain, was likely to work out well. I'm extremely pleased during each visit at how well my analyst is doing. His getting well makes me feel better—like I'm getting well too. It's also reassuring that, if necessary, there is always the telephone from California.

I have no way of knowing what I said or did with Fred and Harriet in those visits except for these letters. I could not take notes and I kept no records of the sessions. I know my speech was a wreck, and that I cut at least one session short because I was too tired. I think I also refused to see him at least once. I know he was considerate of me and would not try to extend a session when I told him I was tiring.

Nine months later, letters indicate he has made a good transition to his new surroundings.

Most of my patients enter into long-term relationships with me which are emotionally significant, and they must have a reasonable conviction that I will be able to function adequately. Since Fred was leaving town, that was no problem for him, but it was for others. It was a problem for Naomi, who put me in this quandary. She had little faith in anyone.

Much of medicine is based upon faith—I had faith in my doctors, and had good reason to. While some sort of faith is necessary, the usual meaning of faith—complete confidence or belief in someone—is not necessary or useful in psychotherapy.

Why should a severely depressed, anxious, or phobic (one who has unreasonable fears) person have faith in a stranger? The patient comes to the doctor scared, but hoping for the best. If he is the kind of person I described, he is guarded or denies his guardedness, at least to himself. Indeed, his basis for embarking upon therapy is hope—because that is all he has—and lack of faith. Faith comes only when the therapist has proven in action that there is reason for it. Naomi writes about "sawing off the limb" and "massive denial." Faith was a hard thing for her to discover.

Naomi

Naomi is a young woman of about thirty-five, with symptoms of severe anxiety and depression. She had the misfortune of undergoing about five years of psychoanalytic therapy with a man who had done little or no good, and certainly never diagnosed the depression she was suffering from.

With great emotional trauma to herself, she broke off her treatment with him and set about to find someone she thought would be better. She went to many people to get lists and ended up with about five names. The first one she went to turned her down because of other duties. I think I was a poor second on the list in her eyes.

It was a tough decision for her and she was constantly testing me. We had worked together for about a year when the stroke hit. Our dilemma was this: she had broken off one relationship and she was gaining confidence in me when I was knocked out of action. She wanted to continue with me, but could I take it? Could I help her?

A bit of Naomi's history is important. She was guilt-ridden, and much of it had to do with enjoying herself. Talented and attractive, she considered herself a failure because she had been a bad child and not made her parents happy. In addition, her younger sister—the only sibling—had killed herself while Naomi was pregnant for the third time, six years ago. Naomi's first recognized panic started a few months after that, and two months before she gave birth. The panic was seemingly brought on during New York City's blackout while she was in a restaurant. Her therapist (George) seemed to feel that he could supply the security she had missed in childhood and thereby reduce her anxiety.

There are some reasons for this. She confided in several people who were, as she said, "reliable" in that they could offer security; she's charming, verbal, and they were her security blanket. The problem was that this was a cover-up for her depression—which stemmed from guilt about her parents, and her hatred (guilt) about feeling that her parents had caused her sister's suicide. After a while, George said, "Stop calling these other people. When you feel panicky, call me." He was frequently unavailable however, because of minor illnesses, and was unable to answer her requests for reassurance.

After my stroke, she wrote me two letters before I saw her. The pertinent parts follow:

Dated 6 days post-stroke

Dear Dr. Dahlberg,

I guess I really know what dependence means now, and it can be pretty hard (but not impossible). The first two days when I knew only that you were "ill," and "in the hospital undergoing tests," were awful, and I think I sobbed more constantly, and harder, than I ever had before. (Not my dramatic verbiage, but really.) Will you tell me when you can, that some of the tears were for my sister? It didn't feel that way. I felt totally deserted, and the only person to whom I needed to tell it, was inaccessible, and was, in fact, the reason I felt that way. I kept remembering your promise to me early on, to try not to saw off the limb I was climbing onto, and when your wife called from the hospital on Friday night, you'd kept the trust.

It struck me, on Thursday evening, that not knowing was the main part of the awful mess, and I screwed up my courage to call Dr. Silver, whose name you'd once mentioned as covering for you. (It was very hard to call him. I don't know why.) Dr. Silver was awfully nice; he told me you'd had an "accident," and once I understood that it didn't mean you'd fallen out of bed, he went on to tell me what good progress you were making and suggested that I call again in a few days for more information.

Most of the sobbing stopped then, and I settled in to wait for word from you or your wife, which came the next night and practically put me back together.

The amazing thing is that I haven't really panicked, or become any more anxious than I'd been (which has been less anxious than in a long time, you know), and I think perhaps it was because I was experiencing all this in such a damn r-r-r-real way! (which perhaps, gruesomely, makes this some kind of positive experience for me). I want now to see you and say it all. I have enough grist for a million mills, but I CAN WAIT.

I think about you an awful lot, and that's not all self-centered. I ache sometimes imagining your feelings, and want very very much for you to be well, for yourself and not only for me.

Nine days after first letter, another letter from Naomi
Dear Dr. Dahlberg,

These last few days have been hard. After my talk with Mrs. Dahlberg from your bedside last Friday, I prepared to wait to hear from her, as we'd agreed when you were home and "seeable." I felt strong enough not to need the support of another "shrink." I guess old "massive denial" was at work because I felt I'd surely hear something within a few days. It seemed a very "cut off" time, and I was quite depressed, but not anxious. By Wednesday, the excitement over Marc's new job was tumultuous, and my concerns about you were approaching panic. On Wednesday night it all exploded into a horrible, weird fit of some kind of hysteria where I lurched around the house, sobbing and screaming in enormous anger about not being able to go through it all again with another doctor, that it wasn't fair, and I was too fucking sick of making all the damn decisions, and why didn't the stinking phone ring? It went on and on until my body suddenly got very, very cold, and I got myself under a couple of quilts and fell asleep.

I guess I was pretty scary, because when I awoke (Thursday) shaken but pretty okay to another day of work and worrying, Marc did a shocking thing. He decided, without telling me, to go to see you in the hospital to find out what was really happening. But you weren't there; you'd gone home, he was told. Surprising news, but good, and now I knew Mrs. Dahlberg would call. Another night of vigil at the phone until Marc persuaded me to call your wife at about ten o'clock.

Our conversion was encouraging, but strange. You were home and asleep, and had mentioned the need to call me and several other patients. She said you were able to talk on the phone (a surprise to me), although your speech was still thick and you sounded a little drunk, (though you weren't—joke!), and your mouth turned down a little at the corner, but it was mending very rapidly. She was sure you'd call back tomorrow or soon! (What the hell did that mean? Sounded ominous.) Well, it obviously wasn't tomorrow, which was yesterday, and now it all feels different. Now I feel angry, neglected, and very impotent. Somehow, you seemed more accessible in the hospital, what with your wife and Dr. Silver. What the hell is "soon" and why? If you aren't ready to speak on the phone, which isn't surprising, why doesn't your wife say so? Are you very, very depressed? Are you planning to cut your patient load, and looking for a good replacement before someone contacts me? I think I could deal with knowing you were unavailable for six weeks or something determinate, but not knowing is very, very hard, and staring at the telephone continuously is becoming impossible. Have I totally lost my perspective?

I called before or after I received the last letter. I don't remember exactly what I said to her when I saw her, but it was something similar to this: "Summertime is coming on and if you start with somebody else now, he'll be going on vacation soon. I don't know if I can help you. I can't write a note to remind myself of what either of us say. My memory is bad. I can try to speak to you, but you can see how hard it is at times. I certainly can't charge you for the kind of work I think I'm doing, but maybe we can help each other a little bit. At least I'll get a chance to find out whether I can think like a therapist. Maybe I can help you." So we agreed and it worked out fairly well.

Naomi realized that it was no time to find another therapist. She remembered with bitterness one of the ones she had called before starting with me. He had told her that since he could not see her very often for a few months, it would be better not to begin after the earlier experience. I understood his reasoning, but that didn't stop her bitterness. But it did make her realize that this would not be a good time for another switch.

I would struggle for words with her, sometimes holding my head in my hands to shut off sight and sounds to get words in proper order. She suffered with me—probably much more than I did.

She was the patient I had seen on my "crazy day"—after two people had recognized my voice on the phone. When I realized how nutty I had been I called her up to tell her. She told me (jokingly) that she thought I was just drunk, but the next day called to say, "I can't save you." My analytic training came to my aid and I told her that that was the beginning of insight: "You don't have to save—can't save—me, your sister, or your parents." Clearly my stroke, and my statement that perhaps we could help each other, played into her problem of having to pay for her guilt by saving people she was angry at.

One of her fantasies had been to have an analyst all to herself. Since she never crossed paths with Fred or any other patient—it was more than enough for me to see one patient on any day—her fantasy was fulfilled. Like many fantasies, the reality was different. Although it was all made to her order— I could see her almost any time she wanted and could stretch the length of the session—she soon wanted the regular order of things. I think she felt she was a burden and didn't want to think about me and my needs. I did try my damndest to stop her efforts to cheer me up. However, it was hard for me to stem her protective instinct; protecting the psychoanalyst interferes with good therapy.

Anita

One of the many interests I have had in the last five years is death and its meaning to the dying and the living. It was part of the research I did with LSD, which is not pertinent here. It did, however, lead to seeing another patient. Few therapists are interested in death; Anita heard of my studies and asked to see me.

Unlike most of my patients, I had known Anita and her husband slightly. She was a friend of Jane's, having taught at the same college a few years back. Her husband had developed brain cancer about a year before she came to see me, and was dying. She asked if I would try to help her work through her difficulties in understanding what was happening to them both, and to help her accept it and treat him as well as possible. I agreed.

I saw her about once every two weeks, although once in a while she would stop coming for a month or so because she didn't want to get too dependent. This was fine. Her husband died about fifteen months after his symptoms started, and about nine months after I began to treat her. He died during the summer after my stroke. Shortly after I had returned from the hospital he called me to "welcome me to the brain damaged." The call was brief—neither of us could talk much, though we could laugh—and I appreciated that he could even think of me with his problems.

Anita is a writer, and I think one can see all that needs to be said from the following:

For several weeks, my discussions with Clay concerned Pete's progressive deterioration and my attitude toward it. I would describe the progress of his illness, discuss the most recent disasters that had befallen him, and, of necessity, spent much time discussing my fears and my dread of the succeeding stages of his illness. It happened that these were the weeks when Pete first began to develop speech problems. I already knew that he definitely and inexorably would be losing his ability to speak. He did not yet know it, or at least we could pretend for the time that we were dealing with a slight deterioration, a weakening of the facial muscles, the lips, the vocal cords. There were as yet no symptoms of aphasia. But Clay and I discussed aphasia and my horror of what this enforced muteness would mean. It seemed to me the worst kind of impairment possible, incomparably worse than the seizures, the paralysis, even the hemiplegia. I always felt it would be the terminal point beyond which there could be no meaningful existence, no communication, no purposeful life. I do not now remember whether I ever said this to Clay in so many words, and I suspect I don't remember because I did say so and feel guilty about it. But I am certain my dread of it must have come across to him strongly. The fact that I have since learned that this fear, like most others, was groundless, is still astonishing, but irrelevant to the particular subject I am discussing. At the time I had certainly no inkling that life, communication, and meaning would go on even beyond this impairment.

Then one day Jane called me and told me Clay had suffered a stroke. He was doing well and would survive and recover, but his face was slightly paralyzed on the right side and his speech was impaired. He was aphasic!

These were Pete's symptoms, the very horrors I had discussed for weeks with Clay. The same side of the brain was damaged. I had a very detailed and graphic awareness of the danger, the potential, and the possibilities for deterioration. I mistrusted the reassuring information made by Clay's doctor to Jane. I had good reason by then to distrust cheerful medical predictions. Jane was telling me all this with a kind of naiveté about what it meant and what it might mean, which struck me as remarkable in so bright a woman. I realized she was unable to face the worst possibilities, so I suppressed my own misgivings. Acting protective toward her gave me something useful to do and say.

I felt terrible for her and terrible for Clay, but I could not then separate it from the all-encompassing private warfare in which I was engaged. With the supreme egotism of a person in a deep personal crisis, everything that happened around me was directly and immediately related to me. It was clear that what had happened had been brought on by me. Death is chasing you, I thought, and he is getting closer and closer. It's the old, vicious cat-and-mouse game.

Some weeks earlier, Mr. E., a neighbor who had visited Pete on Sunday in the best of health, dropped dead of a heart attack on Tuesday. I took that personally, too, but with a wry smile. One down, two to go, I thought, the way my father had always said it. When it rains, it pours. Disasters come in bundles. Three was the magic number. Even more recently, another friend had died of cancer—I had not even told Pete about it yet. So that made two.

After having seen Clay at the hospital I felt more inclined to accept his doctors' prognosis. He would not die; I felt reassured about that. So, I felt death was playing games with Pete and me. That was on the magic level—the childish three-is-the-number level. Although I could easily enough dispose of that, it was strong, nevertheless. Because, after all, I spent night after night in that room holding death at bay by sheer will power; seeing him sitting in the corner, hearing him breathe and whisper. Forcing myself to look him in the eye and say, "Shut up—I'm not afraid of you, so go chase yourself." Which he did, for a time.

But he got hold of Clay, almost, just for kicks, and that's the way it felt to me because there was a jinx on me, and if Clay hadn't gotten involved with us this wouldn't have happened. Perhaps if Mr. E. hadn't come to visit us he'd be alive and well. How can an intelligent woman operate on such a primitive witchcraft-level of feeling?

All of this, while symbolically true, was on the fun-and-games level. In fact, I was feeling horribly guilty about having talked to

Clay as I had, when he now had to live through his symptoms. But the man was a professional, after all, I reasoned. He told me, too, the first time I saw him after his illness, that he could "handle" all this with the proper detachment. I was polite about it then and I appreciated his assurance. I think when he said to me, sharply, with that tone of authority, this is hubris, he was closer to the mark. Yes, it is hubris and it is close to the madness that makes one think one is God, or at least Jesus Christ selected for martyrdom, suffering, and redemption. Very well, and as soon as that was said I could tell myself reasonably—get off it, woman, you know very well you don't cause strokes.

Rationality serves us well, except when we deal with the irrational. I don't cause strokes, and death is not a skeleton sitting in the corner of Pete's room, and the rain dances will not bring us rain. The irrational in our lives has to be accepted without looking for causes. There are no patterns to it. Accidents and coincidences are real. They happen and they have to be accepted. Unfairness, cruelty, and suffering happen randomly and we have to learn to live with that.

On yet another level, I felt cocky as a result of Clay's illness. At least, I thought, I won't have to be a burden to him now. I can pull it alone, which I could and did and which, right away, made me feel reassured about my remaining health, strength, and general ability to cope. Still, I know that in my situation I need help, and I can accept it when I get it. I guess it's no disgrace to be human.

Anita agreed to write the above when I told her about the book. She edited the original, more dramatic version, herself. It came as a surprise—I could not have known what she was going through. I referred her for continuing therapy to a colleague of mine who shared my interest in the problems of the dying.

After leaving the hospital I called all my patients when I was able to speak with some amount of sense, and each was, of course, glad to hear my voice. I set up appointments at intervals with each of them so I could find out what they wanted to do; wait for me to see them when I could, refer them to someone else, or simply stop therapy. It also seemed important that they should have a look at me to see what was actually wrong with me—that I was not a crippled wreck.

They were all grateful for this. Only one, because of other commitments, could not work out a time to see me before I left for Europe.

The patients fell into several categories. Some had to be transferred elsewhere, others said they would wait until the fall and see what would happen then. I was grateful, but also told them that nobody could tell me at what point my recovery might stop, and where I would be then. At that time I had great difficulty in remembering, and I could not write to help my memory. One patient needed a prescription refilled and I had her do it, from my dictation, and I signed it.

One young patient, a former drug addict with whom I had worked for a long time, wrote me a letter. It was cheerful, full of gossip about work, and said at the end, "My parents send their best. If you can have visitors I would like to come in and see you (that is if you don't charge for social calls). Get well soon." I had previously gotten a warm letter from her mother which said, referring to her daughter, "It's so delightful to be able to enjoy her again. We deeply appreciate your part in it."

When Joan came to see me she was trying to be breezy and as she said, "play it cool." She reached the top of the stairs, looked at me, and burst into tears. She hugged me and must have cried for ten minutes on my shoulder before I said, "I guess we'd better go into the office." I don't remember much about the interview, if you can call it that. Then she said "I don't know what would have happened to me if this (the stroke) had happened when I was in the hospital," referring to a time when she went into a deep depression and decided to get off drugs. She had had terrifying experiences and hallucinations and I spent a good deal of time with her.

Two patients at first said they'd see how things went in the fall. One of them said, "I've been seeing you a long time, and much of it was interrupted even before your stroke because I was ill and had two operations. I think I now want to try it by myself." She had not had that recognition until she talked to me. "What do you think about that?" she asked.

I replied, "When my kids wanted to leave home I said,

'Great.' You know you can always come back for a visit or even for a longer time."

"You know," she said, "I never felt that way with my mother. She always seemed to be hanging on." That seemed to be a good conclusion for her.

Of course, many patients were angry—I had let them down. But I believe them when they say that the overwhelming feeling was of sorrow for me.

Some patients, however, did not share the positive feelings about me in general, as expressed in the above comments. One such woman was Linya. She is a petite, attractive woman of about forty. From a small town in the midwest, she had come to New York and made good in the business world. Yet she always felt herself undeserving and was afraid of almost everything. Nevertheless, she persevered, gained some prominence, and although attracted to men, put a wall between herself and them. This was the patient I had not been able to see before I went to Europe because of conflicting schedules.

Dear Clay,

Reactions to your stroke . . .

Upon first learning of your condition, my concern was for you. I was truly fearful of the effect it would have on your life—including your family, your practice, your teaching, and your writing.

It was only after several weeks that I began to question the repercussions of the incident on my own being. I started to wonder about the possible dangers of abrupt, unscheduled termination of therapy on patients in general—and on me in particular. While I did not notice any appreciable differences in my feelings or behavior, I pondered whether this might not be the work of some clever repressing.

However, as the months slipped by and there was still no apparent increased distress (depression, anxiety, etc.), I decided that I did not need to return to therapy. At least not for the time being. (Perhaps this was partially due to an interim method I had adopted for dealing with your unavailability. Whenever I felt I wanted to consult you, I simply did so in my imagination. That is, I pictured you in my mind and then fantasied our conversation.) In any event, since my perceived need for therapy was minimal, I opted for exploring the possibility of 'checking in with you' on an infrequent basis and was relieved to find you agreeable to such an arrangement.

Our first session together was very satisfying to me. You seemed well on your way to total recovery—which made me feel good. Furthermore, you were more open and responsive which permitted me an unprecedented closeness. This, incidentally, was not repeated on my second visit. By that time you seemed to have returned to your cool, aloof self. Pity.

Fondly,
Linya

My work, as I described it earlier, consists of participant observation; listening, watching, remembering, sorting out information, asking questions, and commenting. I must focus on the patient, think about the patient, hypothesize, and apply theories. Empathy, sympathy, patience, knowing when to let the patient ramble on or be silent, when to intervene, what will help or offend—these are some of the therapist's functions. And communication is probably the most important process in the relationship—communication via words, signs, and gestures. Communication that is explicitly clear to the patient, teaching the patient how to communicate better, listening to my own thoughts evoked by the patient's, and recognizing transference and counter-transference are all vital aspects of the therapy process.

The training for psychoanalytic therapy is arduous. It consists not only of studying theory and technique, but also of a great deal of supervision of patient treatment and personal psychoanalysis. The problem is to listen, and to listen with care to all the nuances. This is strenuous, but after a long period of time and experience one gets to the point where remembering every little thing is no longer necessary. At that point one can listen to the patient, to one's own fantasies, and arrive at some kind of "third ear" as described by Theodore Reik. To use a pilot's expression, we are, at that point, "flying by the seat of our pants." We are listening but we are listening in a different mode.

I found that to a large extent that state was gone. I had retained all the tricks: I could associate, I could remember some things, I could pull things together, and I could with hesitation ask a question. I could not count, however, on that special therapist state which years of training and experience provide. Whatever I did required intense concentration and great effort.

The fatigue was bearable for an hour or less. The usual session is a "fifty minute hour," leaving ten minutes between patients to stretch one's legs, make a phone call, write a note, or get some coffee. It amuses me now to remember a paper I once gave at a meeting of pyschoanalysts on "The 100 Minute Hour," in which I cited the advantages of a continuing, uninterrupted longer session, and the need for greater flexibility in allowing the patients more time. I once spent a whole day with one patient, I now can barely last fifty minutes.

Memory is another one of my problems. Not being able to recall all the patient says, not only in one meeting but perhaps five, ten, or fifty sessions back, seriously limits the role of the participant-observer. I could not write at all in the beginning, and even when my writing came back, I still could not write while someone else was talking. If I could have written, it would have been a memory aid for practicing my profession.

One patient, in a state of depression, came to see me shortly before I was leaving town. I felt he should try an antidepressant drug and fortunately I remembered the name. I gave him the prescription pad, dictated the prescription to him, and signed my name. Then I had him write down the same thing for my records. I told him about a possible side effect, whom to call if he needed help while I was away, and when to call me again. As he was leaving my office I asked where he put my copy of the prescription. He was in a bad state and couldn't remember, and I couldn't either. I eventually found it, but that's not the way to practice medicine.

My writing problem was most limiting in my inability to take notes. Why didn't I tape the sessions with the patients? Primarily because tapes have to be typed in order to be useful for memory, and all emotion and nonverbal communication would be lost in the transcript. Transcribing is also costly and time-consuming. In addition, memory is most helpful in therapy when I can respond at the time the issue is raised; tapes or transcripts don't help at that point. Memory has to be currently on tap.

The real problem is that it now requires too much effort to do the many things that once came automatically. It's not a good way to deal with human lives.

Except for an occasional meeting with a former patient, I had to stop my practice for twenty months. I did go to some psychiatric conventions and honored a previous commitment to speak at a symposium in Detroit a year after the stroke. These were at great effort but I thought I had to put in a public appearance once in a while.

I did learn from working with Naomi that I could still think like a psychotherapist. As time went on it got easier.

9

Back Into
the World

Most doctors seem to know very little about the details of prolonged recovery from a severe illness. I suspect that we have enough to do just attending the acutely ill. Once the patient's serious symptoms have passed, medical expertise does not play much of a part. In his busy world the doctor is off and running to the next case. However, it would be helpful to the patient to know about some of the more common complaints he is likely to encounter after the crisis has passed. It is what Sir William Osler meant when he said that "every doctor should have a severe illness and a major operation."

Each patient's recovery is different. The rate of recovery, the specific aches and discomforts, the individual strengths and weaknesses, tensions and concerns are all as variable as our own personalities and individual psychologies.

It's up to the patient to cope with recovery. We set our own pace, and design our new ways of life from one stage of recovery to the next. Adjustments are both physical and psychological. The physical are easier to figure out. For instance, when we returned from Scandinavia in August I was still a cautious invalid. When I went to Leland for a check-up, he noticed my cane and said "Get rid of it." I was to go out, walk vigorously, exercise, and work up a sweat. Since my legs ached all the time, and the more I used them the more they ached, I didn't like this advice, but I followed it and it helped. It was too hot for vigorous walking so we decided on swimming regularly at a nearby pool. I also bought an exercycle—a bicycle that goes nowhere and is about the most boring pastime I can think of. Jane had me set it up in an air-conditioned room in front of the television set, and I now ride several miles a day while watching daytime quiz shows and calculating my mileage (a mind exerciser as well).

I have less energy than I used to and I guess I always will. I must confess that at a party, with a moderate amount of vodka, I find myself dancing, playing, and having fun. I may suffer excessive fatigue the next day, but when I'm not feeling bored and self-pitying, I am much more vigorous.

In fact, we visited some friends on Cape Cod in August and my physical complaints decreased. We had a great time and stayed ten days instead of two or three as planned. Our hosts, Martha and Bill, kept telling us to stay on and I was very happy.

I have had physical symptoms. I am not hypochrondrial (my anxieties take other forms), but after any sort of chronic illness, one tends to look for other things that may be going wrong. I'm sure doctors do this, since they are more aware of what can and sometimes does go wrong: pain in the gut— maybe a cancer which might have caused the stroke; mild aches in the neck—possibly coming from the carotid artery or thyroid gland. Obviously much of this is nonsense, but it happens to you and you have to put up with your own anxieties.

Fatigue continues to plague me, even when I'm enjoying myself. I may suddenly become exhausted and have to excuse myself to take a nap. This is better than boredom and people understand. I've disappeared in the middle of many a social gathering. I tend to be a withdrawn man and Jane is very outgoing. I think that in the long run this is not a bad combination. I keep Jane from wearing herself out with too many social engagements and she keeps me busy with more than I would ordinarily have.

We went to a party recently where I talked with a man

who had had a stroke two years ago. It was particularly
stressful to me because he had, in effect, given up. He had
constant pain in one hand and was consistently depressed.
The meeting with him was a strain and I went home for a
nap. I had a dream about seeing my car abandoned (it looked
like the car I gave my son Johnny). It was left in a careless
fashion because there were still many things of value in it.
The car was being stripped and two tires had been slashed.
The car was me. The dream was set off by meeting this other
man; it must have been about my own feeling of deterioration.

Recovery has been slow since the dramatic improvement of
the early post-stroke days. It seems to get slower every day.
No one can predict the rate of recovery, and each symptom
disappears on its own time schedule. I suddenly noticed, for
example, that only one arm hurt when I was writing. I realized one day that I was picking up short scientific articles
and reading them; soon after I could return to reading more
complicated and better books. I found myself following conversations at a party in a room filled with other people talking. I also was delighted to realize that I had more confidence
in my recovery. I was returning to my old self; correcting
people on points they made, disagreeing about something and
often finding out I was right. No more "stroke personality."

My writing has improved, but is still difficult. I have to sit
down, rest my elbow on the table, and write slowly and
carefully for it to be legible. Writing ability tends to recover
more slowly from aphasia than speaking ability. I can now
edit what I have dictated or written; that is, I can usually see
mistakes. Jane still writes letters and fills out forms (she has
endless energy and patience), and helps with my spelling,
which is slow in coming back. I interrupt her frequently to
ask her how to spell a word, often a simple word. "How do
you spell 'usually?' " "U-s-u-a-l-l-y." "Not so fast." She spells
it again slowly, and then I usually learn the word and hold on
to it. This is in sharp contrast to my status two months after
the stroke when I could not even copy a word when it was
written out for me. My continuing difficulty with spelling

probably has to do with the residual aphasia. It shows up also when I use a dictionary; I still can't find a word easily.

My speech is about back to normal. Other people say they can't notice anything wrong, and I don't get concerned about it except when I am tired. I have learned various strategies to get around missing words, and when I pause to try to find a word people don't seem to notice it because it is a common experience. It used to happen to me prior to the stroke. The more rapid recovery of my speech ability may be because I may have put more emphasis upon, and energy into speaking. I've always been fascinated by words. The brain uses energy, and that part of the brain being exercised uses more energy. In being word-oriented and involved with the derivations of words, I speak more. It may be that I am exercising the language areas of my brain and bringing them back to a more normal state because of that interest. If I were more interested in golf, I might be exercising my arm a great deal more, and bring that ability back sooner.

I have done a lot of complaining about my loss of memory and this warrants some explanation. Some things are remembered clearly and others not at all. This has been true from the very onset of the stroke. I remember some of what went on the first twenty-four hours—things that were very important to me. There was never a problem with visualized events—faces, the hospital, and my home.

I forced myself into compulsive orderliness to avoid losing things. Jane will laugh when I speak of orderliness because my study is a mess, but things which are important to me are in neat piles where I can find them.

Much of what I remember or forget now has to do with emotion. Emotion and retention are hooked up, both positively and negatively. We tend to remember pleasant things, although sometimes we hold on to the unpleasant events. For instance, I can't forget the humiliating incident in the hardware store, shortly after I first went out, when I couldn't remember the name of the item I wanted. Motivation also affects memory. Since I've been writing a book, I wanted to remember the humiliations, frustrations, and angers, as well as the happier moments.

The fear of recurrence is always there and there is no point in denying it. A simple act of adjustment was to start carrying identification cards in my wallet. All my life I avoided carrying credit cards, calling cards, and "what to do in case of emergency" cards in my wallet. Also, I've never been sick, and never imagined that anything would happen to me. In Copenhagen it suddenly occurred to me that if I became ill even if I could talk, I couldn't pronounce the name of the street I lived on (a long Danish name). Jane made out a card for me with all relevant information, and since then I've become a card carrier. Latest cards include: one for donating my eyes to the eye bank in case of death; and a card saying I wear contact lenses which are to be removed if I'm found unconscious. I haven't solved the problem of which cards are most important and should be on top, but I'm covering all emergencies I hope.

Drastic adaptations have to be made to chronic illness, not only by the patient, but by family and friends. It must be clear by now that we are a close family, that Jane especially had to make many adjustments, and made them thoughtfully and with no fuss. I'm sure she is as concerned as I about the possibility of another stroke, and I've taught her and our sons what to do in that eventuality. One simple action, if the symptoms are similar as before, is to lay me down flat on my stomach, turning my face to the side (as you do with a baby); the flatness is for circulation, and being on my stomach prevents me from choking. A more difficult thing to teach Jane is how to inject me with cortisone if a doctor is not available (she's squeamish). This reduces brain swelling until I get to a hospital. She has practiced sticking needles into oranges, and in her efficient way, has written out every step in the process, keeping the list in a handy place.

One can't tell the family what to do under all conditions, when you don't know what's going to happen. What we have done is to talk frankly about the situation, the possibilities, my limitations, and, sometimes, how we feel about it. We don't discuss feelings too often; one can only say one feels depressed, worried, or scared so often—after it's said there is nothing to add. Although I can not say I am sanguine about my future, I don't worry too much about it. I've had no setbacks and I'm functioning.

Psychological recovery and adjustment are not as obvious as the physical—bells don't ring to announce personality changes. Confidence in myself has improved. I travel about the city, argue with shopkeepers, attend professional meetings and speak my mind; I debate politics with my father-in-law, give Jane orders, and now blame the dog when I step on him instead of assuming it was my fault. Maybe I'm less lovable, but it's nice to be me again.

As I've been getting my strength back, I've had recurring dreams, essentially ones of frustration about being cheated and being unprepared. Perhaps I am concerned that I won't be able to do what I want. In one dream, I was in a restaurant getting change for a five-dollar bill when I knew I had given a twenty-dollar bill. I was arguing and getting no satisfaction—just frustration. Another recurring dream has to do with school—a class I didn't attend, homework not done, reports not handed in on time. Clearly, these were all doubts about myself.

Part of what has been going on, since the beginning, is an ambivalence about being taken care of and being my old independent self—caught between playing the child and the master. In fact, neither role was open to me. I had to become independent again, but I would never regain my previous physical strength. I hoped I would regain my mental strength, and subsequent events proved that I did.

Jane needs more companionship than I do, and our Scandanavian trip was hard on her. When we returned, she had to get back to work. About this time I read an essay in *The New York Times* by Corliss Lamont in which he said, "A relative of mine, after her husband retired at age sixty-six and was at home most of the time, remarked to me in some alarm that in her marriage vows she had promised to take him for better or worse, but not for lunch every day." I think that was Jane's dilemma and I can certainly sympathize with it, but it left me on my own.

Jane reflected that for a long time, before leaving for work, she laid out my lunch with specific instructions. It suddenly occurred to her one day to ask me if this was still necessary. I was surprised, but when I thought about it I realized that it was not necessary. She added that "marriage for better or for worse assumes that each will try to be better."

Driving home from Cape Cod in late August, we stopped at a motel and I remarked, "I guess this is as good a time as any to take over. I'll sign us in." This was the first time I resumed my "masculine role." I did it, although the card I filled out looked like it was written by an illiterate drunk. I was reminded of a phrase used by the master of malapropism, Arthur Kober; I felt like "throwing up the sponge."

What I started to give up was my preoccupation with myself. It didn't happen all at once, or even easily. A few days after we were home from the Cape, our former housekeeper whom we all loved very much died from a dreadful, prolonged cancer. Jane and I went to her funeral. My only feeling was relief that Ruby was out of her misery. Jane felt that too, of course, but she also felt a deep loss and mourned for a long while. I may have been too self-preoccupied to grieve.

By the fall, when we were organizing this book, Joe and I and our wives spent a weekend with our friend Ruth Duell, and spent most of the time talking, socializing, and having a good time with many other people. The first night there I had a dream which startled me. I was in a room with a lot of other people and it turned out that many of them (including Joe) had had strokes. I was very disappointed and felt that they were taking it all away from me. By "taking it all away from me" I meant my uniqueness. I guess I've had some clue to this feeling because I know that I talk too much about the stroke, my aphasia, and the book. This has been pointed out to me by several people.

If you feel that much of what you have built is threatened, you try to hold on. Talking about illness is one hell of a bore.

Except for the mild concern of one's family and closest friends, it's a dull subject to everybody except doctors when they discuss it scientifically.

People often tried to reassure me by partaking of my symptoms and in effect, sharing my burden. This was annoying. They said they also could not remember names or words, that they often forgot things, and so forth. Their intention was kind. I would reply, "Yes, but it happened to me suddenly." I soon got over this annoyance because what they were saying is partly true. Many of my aphasic symptoms are exaggerations of what happens around middle age as the natural deterioration of brain cells begins. But their denial of my illness took away my uniqueness.

Essentially, the choice is between living and dying. I never did give much credence to Freud's concept of the death wish in all of us. I opted for life. I think humanity survives, despite all sorts of disasters, because we have a growth motive. That is to say, the need to live, to experience, to continue to grow and learn and be, is a part of life. My life does not only consist of feelings of depression, anger, and apathy, but also of elation, love, and joyousness.

Re-entry into the world means getting back into activities which you can still perform, and finding substitutes for those you cannot. I had to stop being bored and thus boring others.

I do have one advantage over most recovering patients. I have a legitimate reason to talk about my illness in the process of writing this book. I could talk into the dictating machine and then discuss my thoughts with Joe, Ruth, Jane, and Nora. When people asked me what I was doing, I could tell them about the book and some of the details.

I gradually realized that I was regaining skills. I could once again do many things I did in the prestroke days—small chores around the house, errands, a little gardening, and repairs. Jane was grateful for this relief from carrying the whole burden of running the household.

We had been having trouble with our car and were collecting tickets for parking on the wrong side of the street. It had to be moved every day to avoid a ticket. Since we seldom used the car we decided to put it in storage for the winter, and I resolved to do this. Jane, as usual, made the phone calls and arrangements. I had to drive the car up to a garage in the Bronx, and then take the license plates, by subway, to the Motor Vehicle Bureau and return home. Jane's driving directions were specific but I got lost temporarily. The weather was pleasant, I had plenty of time, but my stomach felt increasingly more queasy. When I found the garage everything went smoothly, except that my hand shook as I had to sign a paper. Next, I took the subway to the Motor Vehicle Bureau where a kindly lady routinely handled the forms. I told her I had been sick and didn't need the car; she said it didn't matter and smiled gently. The entire process took about three hours, door to door, and I returned home completely exhausted.

In the past, this might have been an annoying, but not exhausting, way to spend three hours. What should have tipped me off that the day would be difficult was the mental preparation the night before. For hours, in a half-dream state, I hazily planned the necessary steps: "Empty the luggage compartment—Bring registration certificate—Remember license plates—Where is the garage?" Ordinarily, a chore like this is not anxiety-provoking.

This incident describes what I mean by "getting back into the world again." Jane had originally offered to go with me but I saw no reason why her help was required. When I discussed the incident that evening, she replied, "You know I think of you as all right now, but when you tell me this I realize that you're not, and how tough things are." I myself forget the difficulties of trying to return to my old "competent" self from the more-or-less invalid I had become. The part of me that wants to be an invalid and be taken care of is very strong. The part of me that wants to be my old self is both weak and strong. I will make my life more manageable, more evenly paced, and perhaps it will be even richer with more leisure time. I am encouraged that in my newfound, leisurely form of life I have been able to gradually eliminate the high blood pressure medication I was taking; after ten months I was forced to stop it all together in order to avoid low blood pressure. I attribute that to decreasing tension and no overwork. I hope I'm right and can continue this way.

Seven months after the stroke I was due to start teaching my course again. I wanted to teach, I knew the material, and it mattered to me that my colleagues thought of me as recovered. The head of the curriculum committee suggested that one of the younger graduates assist me. This would also test him as a teacher, not an unusual procedure. She didn't say so but I think she was sensitive enough to know that I would be quite nervous and might need help carrying the class. What she didn't know was that I could not read aloud. I could make notes and extemporize from them, but I stumbled very badly if I had to read a passage. My assistant and I worked well together and I was very grateful for his support.

Since everyone knew that I had an aphasic problem, and the course was about psychophysiology, I decided that on the first evening I would clear the air by asking my assistant to read the first few pages of this book, up to the point where I went to the hospital. I stumbled over words when I discussed my subsequent feelings, and continued to do so at times during the semester. The class supplied the words I was searching for. This seemed to be no problem; they did not seem to be embarrassed, nor was I. Teaching the course was an appropriate symbol of having completed my cycle from stroke to recovery; I had returned to the world at the point where I left it. Nevertheless, it was many more months before I could practice my profession.

10

Where Clay is Now

<u>Twenty months after my stroke</u> I was encouraged to, and wanted to, renew my practice. I got a few referrals and called a few patients who had kept in touch with me and wanted to return. It was a small practice and not enough to make a living. I felt I had been home too long and wanted more stimulation from other doctors and different kinds of patients. Psychotherapy patients, although individual, are generally middle class and tend to have similarities, and I was getting tired of too much of the same after twenty-five years of practice. In fact most psychotherapists do other work—as I had done myself with my LSD research.

Joe suggested that I had a special expertise. I was well-trained, had a better than average knowledge of psychiatric drugs, and I knew what it was like to have a stroke and aphasia—and I was quite recovered. I had good qualifications. Zuegma, my neurologist, said I was perhaps unique. I should be good in a <u>rehabilitation unit with aphasic patients.</u>

True, I have certain handicaps: my right wrist still hurts a bit and I write fairly poorly, though if I do it slowly it's legible. I have trouble looking up words but I carry an alphabet with me. My memory is good and I can order my thoughts. My facial drop is unnoticeable except to a doctor who knows I have had a stroke. Because of some problems in speaking and finding certain words I am more than usually vigilant and this creates fatigue.

194

Yet, Joe's idea intrigued me. I talked to friends and had many referrals to rehabilitation and speech therapy centers. I explained I wanted a part time, paying job. Everyone encouraged me and said the world would welcome me. I was breaking new ground. I started making calls, visiting heads of departments, and giving a few lectures on my personal experiences to doctors and nurses. I got nowhere.

No doubt a number of factors were working against me. We were in the middle of a growing economic depression and money was tight. Rehabilitative medicine is largely concerned with the physical aspects of strokes, and while psychological problems are recognized, they have rarely been dealt with by trained psychiatrists. This is, at least in part, the fault of the psychiatrists who have ignored rehabilitation. I also found out that rehabilitative medicine is on the low end of the totem pole in most large hospitals and therefore poorly funded.

Although I aroused interest, there was no offer of pay. Offers for a free consultation and one offer of hospital facilities turned up. I was also told that, "perhaps we could get a grant in the future." But I had to start earning a living, and I was looking for a job at the age of fifty-seven for the first time in my life.

Naturally I was discouraged, but friends continued to encourage me. I still had input problems. Too many things happening at once confused me but I was able to sort them out later. This was no problem in private practice since I have only one patient at a time. Around this time, I became involved in a court trial and was an expert witness which exhausted me, but I managed well.

Clearly, I was uneasy throughout this period, as is reflected in the following dream which recurred in various forms for many months. I had left medical school for a year and was returning. I knew none of my classmates and felt I was way behind them. I couldn't find the classrooms and wasn't sure I knew how to study anymore. This is a common anxiety dream.

Unexpectedly, a close friend came to my rescue. He had been working for a city agency, The Bureau of Child Guidance (BCG), for many years. BCG tries to deal with the many troubled, brain injured, emotionally handicapped, and physically handicapped children within New York's large city school system. Since I had had training in child psychiatry many years back but had given up the practice of it, I was at least qualified on paper. I had thought of working with aphasic children but no opening was available.

With my friend's encouragement, and the knowledge that BCG was hiring, I hesitantly went for an interview and was enthusiastically hired. I was told that under a new ruling classes for the emotionally handicapped had to have a psychiatrist in each school district and they were having trouble getting them.

With fear and trepidation I went to the first school.

I think I should describe the emotionally handicapped children in my second-to-fifth grade classes. Mostly, they solve problems (which are many) by fighting. They curse. They run around the room—frequently on top of the desks. No one starts a fight but fights are frequent. A few are withdrawn and stare into space. Many are depressed. Few come from intact families. All are of at least average intelligence. The classes are in ordinary schools but somewhat segregated.

They are in classes of ten or under with at least two teachers per class, a part time social worker, a psychologist, and me. I had about one hundred children, the social worker, psychologist, and teachers to get to know. I took the job not knowing what I was getting into but as my friend said, "You can always quit."

I got to know about half the staff and children well. I dreamed without anxiety that I was back in school and doing well, and indeed I was. Learning and getting to know new people, problems, and my job was a challenge.

The job was rough: holding fighting kids down, discovering what was going on in the child's home, what teachers' individual problems were, and what the interactions in the classroom were. I have never had so much fun in my life or been as exhausted at the end of the day.

So that's where I am. The job at BCG takes fifteen hours a

week. My family has had to suffer through my stories of the days and the incidents, but they are pleased that I am happy. The principals at the schools expressed their gratitude to me and the rest of the staff at the end of the year. I should add that my blood pressure remained at its normal, prestroke level.

If New York can solve its budgetary troubles I'll retain my job and be back with Mario, Vincent, Jack, and Olga in the fall. Did I say I wouldn't take a rough assignment again? Nonsense. I won't take a dull one!

11

Thoughts for Patients, Families, Friends, and Doctors

1. Patients with chronic illness still have personalities. Fit yours to it. If the patient is obsessively neat, for instance, he will want to remain that way. This is no time to make him change. He has enough to deal with, so allow him to keep what he has.

2. Don't minimize or maximize his symptoms. This is hard, perhaps hardest of all. I restrain my anger when people tell me their memory is slipping too. But also don't invalidize the patient more than necessary.

3. If the patient is a hypochondriac, he will worry and carry on about the most mysterious symptoms—to avoid the anxieties about the real illness.

4. Try to stimulate the patient's interests, perferably in those areas he has always been interested in and can still do. I can only say this from my own personal point of view. The racing form was hard but fun and I had my son to discuss it with me. I read and talked to Joe and he got consultants to

talk to me about things like my math problems and my visual memory. As a doctor, I became fascinated with my symptoms and recovery. I think that interest in your body, if you can remain somewhat objective, is good.

5. For the lazy—perhaps let them be lazy. Some essentially lazy people have been forced to work too hard by circumstances. Enforced laziness can be a great relief—without guilt.

6. Recognize the inevitability of secondary depression. It is hard to put up with, but freely expressing it is the best cure, if only a temporary one. These depressions will pass, with good luck.

7. For the very seriously ill, and those with an imminent fear of death, the family should read *On Death and Dying* by Elizabeth Kubler-Ross. She describes the stages which the dying go through, from denial and isolation, to anger, bargaining, depression, and finally, acceptance and hope.

For me, the real message of Kubler-Ross is that these patients (and others) go through these various emotional phases, and acceptance of their feelings helps. Don't try to analyze them or deny their feelings. Feelings are real, if only temporary, and they should not be forced to enter "into a conspiracy of silence" about what they feel.

I can never thank Leland enough for his honesty both in the hospital and afterward. When I imagine a patient in a teaching hospital, listening to the chief and his interns and residents discussing him as if he were a disease, rather than a person, I shudder.

8. The patient may or may not be of help. If the brain (or other) damage is too great, interest, motivation, energy, and understanding may be beyond him. This is where the ingenuity of the family and friends can help most. Jane and I played what she called charades—sort of a modified version of twenty questions. We did it in five questions. Even the paralyzed patient usually can blink his eyes once for "yes" and twice for "no," if he can understand you. While chronic patients tend to tire easily, they love and need company.

9. For the patient: Mostly, your symptoms are a damned

bore. I had a few doctor friends who seemed interested in mine, but most people were not. My advice is to be straightforward without being tendentious. When asked how you are feeling, answer "Pretty good—improving slowly—but hoping for the best, and expect to be back at work in X number of months."

They really don't want to have an extended discussion of your illness. You will drive them away. I not only learned this myself but Jane told me as well.

Death is an inevitability; don't force people to listen to your woes. They will accept it if you say you are tired and have to rest, but they are not likely to come back soon if you bore them with your sorrows, and you need your friends.